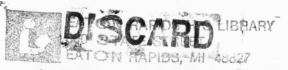

UNDERSTANDING LEUKEMIA

UNDERSTANDING LEUKEMIA

Cynthia P. Margolies
and Kenneth B. McCredie, M.D.

CHARLES SCRIBNER'S SONS · NEW YORK

Library of Congress Cataloging in Publication Data

Margolies, Cynthia P.
  Understanding leukemia.

  Bibliography: p.
  Includes index.
  1. Leukemia.   I. McCredie, Kenneth B.   II. Title.
RC643.M345   1983   616.99'419   83–14110
ISBN 0–684–17978–4

S15704
616.99
MAR
88/89
SHC 13+h
16.95

  3 5 7 9 11 13 15 17 19   F/C   20 18 16 14 12 10 8 6 4

Printed in the United States of America.

CONTENTS

Authors' Notes   vii

1 About Leukemia   1

2 Causes, Coincidences, and Risk Factors
   in the Genesis of Leukemia   27

3 Treatment   78

4 Living with Leukemia   125

5 Research Directions   153

Glossary   199

Sources of Help and Information   225

Further Reading   235

Index   239

AUTHORS' NOTES

The word "leukemia" conjures up an image that is dreadful, that makes many of us want to look the other way. Some of us cannot look the other way—those who are leukemia patients, parents of leukemic children, or who are otherwise personally concerned with the fight against leukemia. There are others who do not want to look away, who want to help in an informed way, or who simply want to know about leukemia—this enemy that could be yours or mine.

Understanding Leukemia is written with the knowledge that some casual readers, particularly those without a fairly firm background in biological sciences or with only a smattering of medically related information, may find the presentation somewhat difficult or too detailed. You who are living in the shadow of leukemia are also likely to find at least portions of the book difficult to grasp, even though you are highly motivated to understand. I would rather tell you more than you may want to know about leukemia, and let you select what is of personal importance. It may seem like forcing you to master a foreign language, when all you want is to get out of that country safely. But you can learn what is being said in the awesome language of leukemia, and how scientists are listening to it, translating it, and preparing answers that can stifle it.

This book is objective; by that I mean I haven't softened certain hard facts. You will find here much important information about leukemia; however, present knowledge may not provide the answers you might wish. I hope that if you want to, or need to, understand leukemia, this book will help.

Cynthia P. Margolies

Medical scientists do not fully understand why leukemia happens. How leukemia behaves is better understood, and this understanding has permitted us the significant advances of recent years in controlling the disease. It is the intention of *Understanding Leukemia* to guide the reader along the paths taken by researchers and physicians in their attempts to find the biological logic that underlies leukemia; the "method in its madness" will give us the key to leukemia's conquest.

In some instances in the history of medicine, particularly in the early days, treatments and remedies for diseases came out of good hunches, trial and error, and happy accidents, with little understanding as to why something worked when it did. In the case of leukemia, it has been necessary to build toward successful treatment with many small blocks of biological knowledge. With the tremendous enlightenment that has come with our increasing ability to view or deduce the microscopic world, we are daily decoding the ways of the sabotaged cells that are called leukemic. We are better equipped to design treatments that eradicate leukemic cells while sparing and strengthening healthy cells.

Today we can offer realistic hope for lengthy remissions and even probable cures for many leukemia patients, something that was not likely even ten years ago. We are optimistic, with reason, that leukemia will soon be conquered. I want to share with the reader many of the reasons for this optimism.

Kenneth B. McCredie, M.D.

Vice President, Medical
and Scientific Affairs,
Leukemia Society of America
and
Professor of Medicine
Chief, Leukemia Service
University of Texas System Cancer Center,
M. D. Anderson Hospital
and Tumor Institute, Houston

CHAPTER ONE

ABOUT LEUKEMIA

Leukemia, a term derived from the Greek, literally means "white blood." It was coined in 1847 by a German doctor to describe a disease in which the blood was overrun with white blood cells. As medical science now knows, "white blood" is apparent in only about half of the cases of leukemia, and the disease is rooted not in the blood itself, but in the blood-forming tissues.

Until the 1960s, there was no effective treatment for leukemia. The acute forms usually killed within months, while individuals with the chronic forms might survive several years. There is now, at long last, optimistic news about this dread disease—a disease never more devastating than when it claims the life of a young child.

Today the most common type of childhood leukemia is potentially curable in about 60 percent of cases. This means that 60 percent of young patients will survive at least five years, a milestone considered by many physicians to indicate probable cure.

The adult types of leukemia are more resistant to treatment, and the survival rate of those stricken is lower than that of children. However, there are now increasing numbers of reports on successful disease management—lives extending beyond the five-year marker—among adult leukemia patients.

There are an estimated 24,000 new cases of leukemia in the United States each year. About 16,000 Americans die from the disease each year, accounting for 9 percent of all deaths due to cancer. Although it is often considered a disease of childhood or adolescence, in fact, leukemia strikes many more adults—21,500 each year, compared to 2,500 children. More than half of all cases of leukemia occur in persons over sixty.

Unfortunately, there is nothing simple about understanding leukemia. Some of the material in this chapter may seem better suited to a medical school course or an advanced biology class. But we feel that this completeness is necessary, in order for you to understand the complexity of the disease and the reasons behind the methods of treatment. Whether you are a leukemia patient, the parent of a leukemic child, or a general reader with interest in medical topics, you need to be introduced to the basics of cancer in general, relevant cell biology, the leukemic process, and types of leukemia. We have tried to present this material as clearly and simply as possible.

CANCER AS ABNORMAL CELL BEHAVIOR

Cancer, or malignancy, is characterized by an uncontrolled growth and spread of abnormal cells. The basic living units that make up all parts of the body, cells normally reproduce themselves in an orderly manner so that growth occurs, necessary functions are performed, injured tissues repaired, and worn-out or otherwise deficient cells replaced.

The normal cell is highly complex, yet functions with orderliness and efficiency, capable of self-limitation (not taking in more nutrients than it needs, for example) and fine-tuned collaboration with neighboring cells. An individual cell coordinates a wide range of biological activities based on an elaborate communications system and a single goal, survival. Uncoordinated activities on the part of cells—that is, departures from their precise roles and particular "scripts"—invariably lead to pathological conditions. Such wayward cells usually die or are inactivated or killed by the body's defense system.

A normal cell is programmed to coordinate its own objectives, notably to move smoothly through stages of maturity to become fully functional. The cell goes through a process of acquiring traits that will make it a "specialist," a process known by the biological term differentiation. A cell differentiates according to the genetic programming given it by its parent cell, and in response

2

to body chemistry factors that influence its development. The parental genetic programming of a cell gives it in effect a script that defines its organ or tissue location (e.g., skin, lungs, blood), its activities, and what it can become.

A normal cell recognizes its boundaries of structure, activity, and location. Each cell must also act in harmony with neighboring or joint-responsibility cells, sending and receiving chemical messages that signal biological steps.

Malignant cells lack such internal regulation and the capacity for desirable communal activity or reactivity. They are often immature in form, or may be mature "functional illiterates." They may roam and maraud, disregarding obligations and territorial claims.

Although every tissue and organ of the body maintains a "baby bank"—a small group of immature and undifferentiated cells to ensure repopulation when needed—the tissue or organ must be predominantly composed of mature cells or it loses its ability to function. Malignant cells have lost the pages of their script that lead them into productive maturity—that is, their genetic programming has been disrupted.

Malignant cells do little but multiply; and in large numbers they disrupt and can destroy vital bodily processes. Malignant liver tissue, for example, does not provide bile or break down sugars, two functions necessary for life.

Malignant cells can grow into a mass called a tumor, and can invade and destroy nearby normal tissue. They can migrate, in a process called metastasis, spreading via the blood or lymph to other parts of the body. For example, an undifferentiated malignant liver cell, breaking away and traveling, can requisition the same passive hospitality in other parts of the body—and multiply there, as it did in the liver.

What causes normal tissue to begin producing malignant cells? The answer to this question is being unraveled through investigations into the "command post" of the cell, its nucleus, and into the ways and means of the body's immune-response, or self-defense, system. The current status of these investigations will be covered in later chapters.

LEUKEMIA AS A FORM OF CANCER

Leukemia is doubly sinister in that it is a malignant aberration that also strikes at the heart of the body's internal peacekeeping, alien-repelling apparatus. It cripples the commanders of the early-warning immune response, or the soldiers of the immune system (this system will be more thoroughly described in chapter 2). These commanders and soldiers are white blood cells, normally responsible for ridding the body of any malignant cells as well as disease-causing substances and foreign or defective cells.

Leukemia arises in one of the blood-producing tissues, that is, in the bone marrow or spleen; or in the thymus or lymph nodes, way stations and "training centers" for lymphocytes, one variety of white blood cell.

Leukemia is a systemic cancer in that the bodily systems that it affects directly (blood and lymph systems) have access to all the organs and tissues of the body. In its natural course, leukemia will at some point affect all of the blood-forming tissues, the circulatory systems, and the body as a whole.

Leukemic cells are not merely immature or poorly functioning cells; they are nonfunctional cells that take over, becoming the predominant cell type in the circulatory systems, colonizing in organs such as the brain, and inhibiting the generation of normal and vital blood cells. Whatever their point of origin or state of maturity, or wherever their chief haven at the time of discovery (e.g., lymph nodes, spleen), leukemic cells will be manifest in the bone marrow—the spongy meshwork of tissue that fills up the cavities of bones. They will show up in the bone marrow either because they are proliferating and "backlogging" there or because they have migrated back.

THE BLOOD AND LYMPH SYSTEMS

The blood, which contains more than a hundred components, is of vital importance to all cells of the human body; it supplies them with the food, oxygen, hormones, and many other chemicals they must have to function. The blood system, through its arteries, veins, and capillaries, transports these many substances to and from storage centers in various tissues; helps in the removal of waste products; and marshals a formidable defense against defective cells and foreign invaders such as bacteria, fungi, and viruses. The cellular components of the blood are red blood cells (known also as erythrocytes), white blood cells (collectively termed leucocytes), and platelets; the fluid portion of the blood, called serum or plasma, serves as the transport medium and contains important proteins, nutrients, and processing chemicals.

Most blood cells are produced in the bone marrow (perhaps 2 percent are produced in the spleen). As they mature, they are released into the blood at a fairly regular rate consistent with the death rate of old cells. They may be formed and released at a more rapid rate when bodily monitoring and feedback mechanisms send chemical alarm signals to the marrow. Such signals can be given off, for example, when bodily oxygen is low, calling for more red blood cells; or when white blood cells are attacking an infection, calling for more white cells to be formed to serve as back-up troops or combatants.

In humans the various blood cells exist in recognized, normal proportions, both within the compartments of the bone marrow, where they are in a generative or immature stage, and in the blood itself, where they are in a formative or fully mature stage. Many events or intrusions can upset this proportional balance, including toxic substances, infections, hormonal imbalances, genetic deficiences, and faulty signals given by certain cells, such as those that may be malignant, transformed by disease-causing microorganisms, or defective in other ways.

The lymph system, a circulatory system adjunct to the blood system, consists of a connecting network of glands (lymph nodes) and vessels that carry the usually transparent fluid, lymph. The lymph system can be described as a waste-collecting, filtering, and drainage system that extends throughout the body. The vessels of the lymph system are much finer and more delicate than blood vessels. The lymph fluid has ready access to the bloodstream, sometimes by oozing into the tiny capillaries, but particularly through its vessel juncture with the blood system at the thoracic duct, where it can empty into veins.

The blood and lymph systems are illustrated in Figure 1.

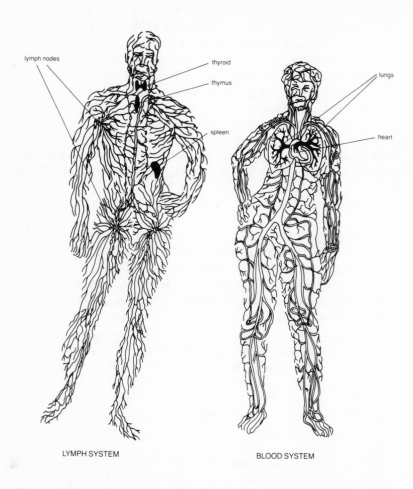

Figure 1. Schematic drawings of the lymph and blood systems. (*Paul Zuckerman*)

BLOOD CELL DEVELOPMENT AND ACTIVITIES

In man, most tissues are made up primarily of differentiated or mature cells that normally show little evidence of proliferation and self-renewal; that is, proportionately few cells are dividing at any given time. The blood-forming tissues, however, along with the skin and the mucous membranes lining the gastrointestinal system, continuously renew themselves. In all tissues a small number of stem, or progenitor, cells divide and differentiate; the more mature cells are derived from these stem cells. Blood cells expend themselves continuously, and their stem pools are constantly active.

Medical scientists now believe that all types of blood cells are derived from a common ancestor, called a pluripotent stem cell, and that this cell originates in the bone marrow. This original progenitor cell can renew itself, through division, and can also produce a more specialized progeny, a parent stem cell that will further develop along one of two distinct pathways; the parent stem cell can also duplicate itself at this stage, through another division.

In appearance, stem cells resemble young lymphocytes (a type of leukocyte); but in laboratory testing they lack certain structural, chemical, and immune-activity characteristics that mark the predominate lymphocyte population. With present techniques (other than waiting to see, in the laboratory, what colonies of cells they will generate), however, stem cells are indistinguishable from cells known as "null" lymphocytes—primitive and undifferentiated lymphocytes. It is estimated that stem cells normally make up no more than 5 percent of cells in the marrow, and considerably less than 1 percent of cells in the blood.

Stem cells can readily migrate, and research has shown that oxygen depletion, anemia, and influx of certain toxins or antigens decrease the marrow supply of stem cells and increase the blood and spleen concentrations of stem cells. Conversely, depletion of stem cells in the marrow induces the stem cells in the blood to travel to the marrow and busily reproduce themselves.

One parent stem cell along with its various developmental-stage versions of itself is called the myeloid line; it includes the cells that will become red blood cells, platelets, and the white blood cells called granulocytes, monocytes, and macrophages. The other parent stem cell together with its descendant cells is known as the lymphoid line, which gives rise to the highly sophisticated white blood cells known as lymphocytes (see Figure 2).

Erythrocytes (Red Blood Cells)

In the development of a red blood cell, the parent myeloid stem cell is influenced principally by need: lack of oxygen in the body (even a slight decrease) is sensed by the kidneys, which produce a hormone, erythropoietin, that stimulates the proliferation and differentiation of red blood cells.

The red blood cells carry the oxygen necessary for life to all the organs and tissues of the body. To do this, each cell contains a small amount of a compound called hemoglobin, which is capable of taking up oxygen as the blood passes through the lungs, and releasing it in other bodily tissues. After delivering its supply of oxygen, the depleted red blood cell returns through the veins and picks up a fresh supply of oxygen from the lungs.

The structure (no nucleus) and functions of red blood cells are quite simple, in cellular terms. Other than their obvious significance in maintaining vigor in an individual through transport of oxygen and prevention of anemia, red blood cells are not of major conceptual importance in relation to leukemia in that they are not part of the immune-response system.

Megakaryocytes (Producers of Platelets)

Derived from a myeloid stem cell, the large megakaryocytes are cells with a distinctive many-lobed nucleus. Megakaryocytes do not circulate in the blood; they remain in the marrow, and the small disc-like platelets break off from them and enter the bloodstream. Platelets are essential for the prevention of abnormal bleeding; they congregate at rupture or trauma sites, clumping together to enable coagulation or clotting. Platelets also participate in an inflammatory response (e.g., to an infectious microorganism) by releasing an active substance called serotonin; this substance causes blood vessel walls to stretch and become more porous,

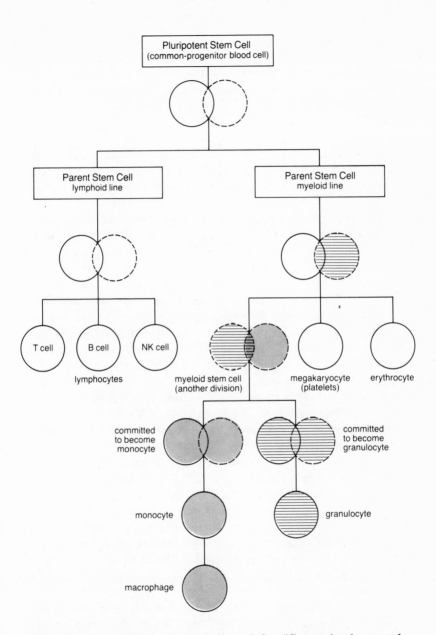

Figure 2. Diagrammatic representation of the different developmental pathways that may be taken by the progeny of a pluripotent blood stem cell (and its self-copies). One cell (hatch marks) differentiates and matures to become a granulocyte; another cell (shaded), to become first a monocyte, then a macrophage. The broken-line cells indicate self-copies, reproduction of a cell through division. *(Harvey Offenhartz, Inc.)*

making it easier for infection-fighting white blood cells to pass through vessel walls and pursue pathogens into nearby tissues.

Leukocytes

Leukocytes are composed of the myeloid line (granulocytes, monocytes, and macrophages) and the lymphoid line (lymphocytes).

The kinds of blood cells can be distinguished from one another by a variety of techniques. It has long been easy to distinguish red cells, white cells, and platelets in a blood sample under the microscope. However, it has proved a long and difficult undertaking for scientists to pigeon-hole the types and subtypes of white blood cells and their various stages of development or differentiation. It is of great importance, in evaluating leukemia patients, to correctly identify the malignant white cell type that is uncontrollably multiplying—its lineage (myeloid or lymphoid), its subtype, in cases of lymphocytic (affecting lymphocytes) leukemia, and its stage of differentiation.

Microscopic examination of white blood cells has proven to be a very inexact means of identification. It has been learned that lymphocytes, monocytes, and macrophages can drastically change their size and the makeup of their nucleus, can change their chemistry, surface structures, activities, and products—depending not only on their stage of differentiation, but also on whether they are quiescent or stimulated, as by an infection or trauma.

Methods of distinguishing white blood cells still include physical techniques, such as studying the appearance of the nucleus and the cytoplasm, and techniques of cell separation, as by weight or density. Additional techniques used in the laboratory to characterize white blood cells now include observing their response to various antagonists and stimulants; introducing other substances that the cell will ignore or bind to itself; looking for characteristic surface or cytoplasm structures that declare themselves upon reactivity-testing; and testing their levels of, and response to, certain enzymes.

Myeloid White Blood Cells: Granulocytes, Monocytes, and Macrophages

The white blood cells of the myeloid line, known collectively as phagocytes, are normally about three times more numerous in circulation than those of the lymphoid line. Normally the type of white blood cells known as granulocytes are the most numerous among the myeloid white cells. Granulocytes, macrophages, and, to a lesser degree, monocytes, fulfill the vital function of ridding the body of bacteria, viruses, and other pathogens; foreign or defective cells (including malignant cells); and smaller foreign or defective organic structures such as proteins.

They perform this scavenging activity by a process called phagocytosis, in which they engulf, ingest, and destroy offending structures and organisms—not only in the blood and lymph systems, but in nearby tissues as well. Phagocytosis is the major *implementation* of an immune response; but most often the myeloid white blood cells must receive an array of stimulatory and guiding signals from lymphocytes—signals that include target-binding (combining with the offensive cell or structure) by some lymphocytes and their products, and corroborating chemical alarm signals released into the blood by various other cells as well. Phagocytosis, which can be demonstrated by reactivity tests in the laboratory, is one principal distinction that sets apart even quite immature granulocytes, monocytes, and macrophages from lymphocytes for purposes of identification.

The generation and differentiation of granulocytes, monocytes, and macrophages from myeloid stem cells are stimulated by loss of mature cells, the presence in the blood of the chemical alarm substances related to an immune response, and certain positive-feedback, or stimulatory, chemicals released into the blood by the activated phagocytes themselves.

Circulating, mature granulocytes respond quickly to the presence of pathogens in or near the bloodstream—pathogens whose presence has been signaled by attachment of the lymphocyte products known as antibodies (to be discussed more thoroughly in chapter 2), and concentrations of other inflammatory stimuli. Granulocytes have a rapid turnover rate and a high volume of production.

11

Their life is often less than a day; and they "sacrifice" themselves, dying upon ingestion and destruction of pathogens.

Monocytes resemble lymphocytes in appearance, but are distinguished by their phagocytic activity and other laboratory "markers." They produce certain biologically active substances, including a hormone, that are important in regulating myeloid stem cells. However, monocytes may best be described as cells in transition; they only circulate in the blood for a few days, then they differentiate into macrophages.

Macrophages are large phagocytes that are generated in the bone marrow by myeloid stem cells, and are released into the blood as monocytes. Their maturation is varied. A portion of them circulate in the blood and lymph, and when not activated they tend to cling to blood vessel walls or to lie dormant in the lymph nodes or the spleen—waiting for lymphocyte signals to lead them to foreign or deficient structures in the circulatory systems. Other macrophages will leave the circulatory systems and take up residence in the liver, the central nervous system, or the lungs, where they differentiate and remain on call.

Until recently, macrophages were viewed primarily as important but unsophisticated scavenger cells, gobbling up debris or offensive ("not-self") chemical structures that were pointed out to them by lymphocytes or concentrations of trail-blazing molecules (the alarm signals mentioned earlier; usually special proteins) released by lymphocytes and certain other cells that participate in an immune response. Studies over the past several years, however, have pointed up the importance of the macrophages' secretions, and their critical role in the immune response and the defense against malignant cells.

Macrophages produce enzymes, contained in internal pockets, that enable them to digest (although not always completely) pathogens, foreign cells, and other biological debris. (Enzymes are a type of protein needed to catalyze biochemical reactions; they control the steps and the rate of a cell's processes—whether the work involves building up, conversion, decomposition, or maintenance and repair.) It has been found that macrophages release fragments of engulfed substances continuously for long periods of time—harmless bits that, it is believed, "teach" lymphocytes to be on the lookout for organisms or biological structures bearing molecules like those released by the macrophage.

Recent investigations demonstrate that the macrophage processes and secretes many highly potent substances that can affect tissue repair and reorganization; lymphocyte recognition of foreign substances known as antigens bearing "not-self" surface markers; lymphocyte proliferation and differentiation; and the suppression of malignant cell growth. Recent work at New York City's Memorial Sloan-Kettering Cancer Center suggests that it is the macrophages' production of the hormones known as prostaglandins that may inhibit malignant cells. Other important secretions of the macrophage include proteins known by the group term "complement"— partners that join with antibodies to bind, and thereby flag, antigen-bearing substances; and interferon, known to suppress virus activity within cells and possibly to inhibit malignant cells.

Lymphoid White Blood Cells: The Lymphocytes

From the lymphoid stem cell's line of differentiated cells come at least three types of lymphocytes. Essentially, the lymphocytes patrol the blood and lymph systems and lymphoid organs (e.g., spleen, thymus, thyroid, lymph nodes), and interdependently identify and attack antigen-bearing substances—including tissue and organ transplants from other persons. Lymphocytes also communicate and interact with the phagocytic white blood cells.

The most numerous among the lymphocytes—75 to 80 percent —are those known as T cells, and they are an exception to the general rule that normal blood cells are mature before being released from the bone marrow. T cells leave the bone marrow in an immature stage and set off for the thymus gland, like newborn turtles heading for the sea. Through stimulatory signals received by cells in the thymus, the immature T cell goes through a developmental period, then enters the bloodstream as a mature and highly specialized cell. A T cell, is thus a thymus-derived lymphocyte.

T cells are believed to be instrumental in initiating an immune response against more complex foreign or aberrant structures found in the body; they are especially attracted to offensive (e.g., foreign or defective) proteins, and particularly those displayed on cell surfaces. For this reason, they are critical to the surveillance of malignant cells, because such cells usually display on their surfaces faulty proteins that are the result of their abnormal internal activities. T cells have special receptors on their surfaces that allow them to recognize a faulty protein or protein arrangement on a suspect cell.

A T cell that has thus recognized an enemy may then perform a number of immune-response activities, depending upon its specific differentiation capability as determined by its genetic programming, its schooling in the thymus, and any know-how acquired in previous encounters with aberrant substances. The T cell may directly bind to the offensive structure on a target cell and transfer chemicals into or out of it, fatally disrupting the target's equilibrium; be stimulated to divide again and again, proliferating into a clone (self-copy) of activated cells; release chemicals that will attract macrophages and other lymphocytes to the scene or release chemicals that will stimulate the differentiation of more young lymphocytes as well as the differentiation of monocytes into macrophages.

Next in quantity among the lymphocytes are those known as B cells, which normally make up 10 to 20 percent of the lymphocyte population. B cells (bone-marrow-derived lymphocytes) undergo their formative period in the bone marrow and are released into the bloodstream with a capability of binding foreign or aberrant structures; but, unlike T cells, B cells have surface receptors that allow them to engage or recognize only a portion of a large offensive molecule (such as a protein), or tiny scraps or particles of undesirable substances.

Once bound to a fragment or portion of an offending structure, the B cell's most significant immune-response capability can come into play. If the attraction between the B cell's receptors and the invading antagonist is strong—if the genetically determined fit is right—the B cell will be stimulated to proliferate into a clone colony of activated cells; some of these will differentiate further, becoming so-called plasma cells, which can secrete antibodies that will seek out and bind to antigens exactly like the original antagonist.

Although any given B cell can generate only one particular antibody, it can secrete this antibody in quantities, and pass on the "formula" to its daughter cells. This is the nature of the body's "memory" for certain infectious agents—the basis of immunities and vaccinations. Antibodies clinging to their antagonists are a stimulus for other participants in an immune response: they attract phagocytes and T cells, and spur the synthesis of chemical-alarm molecules by those cells as well as others.

Less than 5 percent of an individual's lymphocytes are of a type only recently recognized as distinct from T and B cells. Called "natural killer" lymphocytes (NK cells), these cells appear to have the ability to kill malignant or virus-infected cells on contact and without the interactions that typify immune-response sequences. They also have the astonishing ability to kill foreign cells without previous exposure to them.

The NK cell's role in surveillance of and attack upon aberrant cells—and particularly its role in destroying malignant cells—is under intensive investigation. Its effectiveness appears to be genetically determined.

The lymphocytes often do battle with infectious agents in the lymph nodes, which serve as entrapment sites. Other lymphoid organs (e.g., tonsils, adenoids) also can serve as way stations for lymphocytes, and pathogens can be localized there for destruction. Lymphoid tissue—that is, tissue composed largely of lymphocytes—of other organs, such as portions of the gastrointestinal system, also serve this confinement purpose; in the course of severe infection or chronic inflammation, lymphocytes will congregate in a wide range of nonlymphoid structures, such as the lungs.

OVERVIEW OF LEUKEMIA

It is now accepted that leukemic cells are clones of a few abnormal white blood cells—or very possibly only one abnormal cell—and are not, as mentioned earlier, merely inadequately functioning cells. It is believed also that there is an initial, priming situation or event that produces this cell line, probably preceding overt disease by months or even several years. Most scientists believe that for a cluster of abnormal cells to extend into a significant malignancy, a further deficiency must exist in the individual, or an additional, triggering event must occur. This two-step theory of cancer will be discussed in chapter 2.

Once established, leukemic cells accumulate in the bone marrow, sometimes "frozen" in a very immature state, sometimes in a stage of maturation all but indistinguishable under the microscope from that of normal cells. Leukemic cells continue to divide—although usually not rapidly, as was commonly thought, once the disease is advanced enough to measure. They eventually "spill over" into the blood, and can then be carried throughout the body.

The proliferation of leukemic cells in the bone marrow will interfere with the production of normal red blood cells, white blood cells, and platelets—partly by crowding out normal stem cells and their progeny. In addition, however, medical scientists believe that further suppressive action is present: that leukemic cells possess a structure, or "marker," that inhibits normal stem cells, or else lack a marker that would usually stimulate such cells. An alternative explanation is that, in some types of leukemia, the progenitor, pluripotent stem cell may be the abnormal cell, and that all the descendants of its line, red cells and platelets as well as white cells, are thus defective.

Malignant-cell colonization and proliferation anywhere in the body represent a failure of the immune-response system: the abnormal cells are successfully camouflaged, or there are significant flaws or deficiencies in some components of the immune system. Leukemia is a manifestation of this failure, which is made more extreme by the fact that those cells that are supposed to provide the solution are largely those that are the problem. It is like mounting an attack with troops of saboteurs.

Most Common Types

Leukemia can appear in either acute, rapidly growing forms or in chronic, slowly progressing forms. The acute forms represent the proliferation of cells "frozen" in an immature state; the chronic forms represent a malignant cell population mature in form but not function, which divides slowly.

The types of leukemia (see Table 1), are categorized according to the predominant abnormal cell population: by identification of the parent line (myeloid or lymphoid) if the cell is very immature; and by the cell type and developmental stage as determined by various structural, productivity, functional, and chemical characteristics, revealed upon cell-sample analysis in the laboratory.

TABLE 1. CLASSIFICATION OF THE LEUKEMIAS

COMMON TYPES

ACUTE LYMPHOCYTIC LEUKEMIA (also called acute lymphoblastic, lymphatic, or lymphogenous leukemia): The most common type of leukemia in children; exhibiting a predominant proliferation, in about 75 percent of cases, of extremely immature lymphoid cells that are nonetheless recognizable as cells of the lymphocyte line. In the remainder of cases, the predominant malignant cell population exhibits differentiation markers of either B lymphocyte or T lymphocyte development; but the cells are still at an immature level.

CHRONIC LYMPHOCYTIC LEUKEMIA (also called chronic lymphatic, lymphogenous, or lymphoid leukemia): A slowly progressing malignancy, which in the vast majority of cases is represented by a proliferating clone of fairly mature lymphocytes of the type known as B cells; its highest incidence is in elderly males.

ACUTE MYELOCYTIC LEUKEMIA (also called acute myeloblastic, myelogenous, or granulocytic leukemia): Characterized by a predominant malignant cell population of grossly immature granulocytes or a primitive progeny of a myeloid stem cell insufficiently differentiated to be considered a granulocyte; it occurs primarily in older adults.

CHRONIC MYELOCYTIC LEUKEMIA (also called chronic myelogenous, granulocytic, or myeloid leukemia): A malignancy that originates in a myeloid stem cell, but is manifest in aberrant granulocytes, which, although they may mature, remain incompletely functional and continue to multiply; it is primarily found in older adults. The disease is identified by a specific genetic defect, called the "Philadelphia chromosome," which is apparent in affected cells of the erythrocyte, megakaryocyte, and monocyte-macrophage lines of myeloid cell differentiation as well as the granulocyte line.

LESS COMMON TYPES

ALEUKEMIC LEUKEMIA: A type in which there are not recognizably abnormal white blood cells, but there is a marked deficiency of all blood cell types.

BASOPHILIC or MAST CELL LEUKEMIA: A type in which the predominant malignant cell population is made up of basophils, a subtype of granulocyte that is unique among white blood cells in its capacity to release histamine, an important mediator of an immune response; and/or is made up of mast cells, which similarly secrete histamine, but are tissue cells near the capillaries, not blood cells.

EOSINOPHILIC LEUKEMIA: A type in which the predominant malignant cell population is made up of eosinophils, a subtype of granulocyte that is strongly attracted to certain secreted substances which mediate an immune response.

ERYTHROLEUKEMIA (also called DiGuglielmo's disease): A type in which the predominant malignant cell population is made up of an intermediate-stage stem cell that is committed to develop into a red blood cell; the disease also often involves the proliferation of abnormal cells all along the myeloid line of cell development, so erythroleukemia may well originate in a myeloid stem cell.

HAIRY-CELL LEUKEMIA: A type in which the predominant malignant cell population is made up of an unusual-appearing cell that exhibits tentacle-like projections and is of uncertain derivation—although many scientists believe it to be an aberrant B lymphocyte; the leukemic cells tend to aggregate in the spleen.

MEGAKARYOCYTIC LEUKEMIA: A type in which the predominant malignant cell population is made up of abnormal megakaryocytes, resulting in defective platelets.

MIXED-CELL LEUKEMIA: A catchall category in which several or many blood cell types are abnormal, and in which there is no clearly predominant clone of cells; it is likely that more than one cell line has been malignantly transformed.

MONOCYTIC or HISTOCYTIC LEUKEMIA: An imprecise category in which the malignant cell type is of uncertain origins, resembling both an immature monocyte and an undifferentiated lymphocyte.

MONOCYTIC LEUKEMIA, SCHILLING TYPE: The so-called "true" monocytic leukemia, characterized by a predominant malignant cell type which is an immature monocyte.

MYELOMONOCYTIC LEUKEMIA: A type in which the predominant malignant cell population is made up of intermediate-stage progeny of a myeloid stem cell that shows the beginnings of differentiation along the monocyte line of development.

NEUTROPHILIC LEUKEMIA: A type in which the predominant malignant cell population is made up of granulocytes of the most prevalent subtype—known as neutrophils.

PLASMA-CELL LEUKEMIA: A type in which the predominant

malignant cell population is made up of fully differentiated B cells that have been stimulated to produce antibodies; in this disease the plasma cells are clonal, and produce quantities of a single type of antibody.

POLYMORPHOCYTIC LEUKEMIA: An imprecise category in which the malignant cells seem to change their appearance and their characteristics, with particular confusion among lymphocytes, monocytes, and macrophages.

PROMYELOCYTIC LEUKEMIA: A type in which the findings suggest myelocytic leukemia, but the abnormal cells are extremely primitive; other factors that could determine myelocytic leukemia may also be dubious.

RIEDER CELL LEUKEMIA: A type in which the predominant malignant cell population is made up of immature myeloid cells that exhibit deep indentations of the cytoplasm into the nucleus, indicative of disparity in age between the nucleus and cytoplasm; the distorted appearance is marked.

STEM-CELL LEUKEMIA (also known as embryonal leukemia, although the term is largely obsolete): A category in which the malignant cells can be recognized as stem cells because of their primitive development and their ability to generate, upon stimulation in the laboratory, clusters of more differentiated progeny, rather than simply duplicates of themselves.

UNDIFFERENTIATED LEUKEMIA (also called "null" cell leukemia): A category in which the malignant cells do not exhibit distinctive differentiation markers that would identify their developmental destiny; yet they often exhibit enzyme activity that can be the basis for at least identifying their lineage as lymphoid or myeloid.

In the United States, the most common type of leukemia in children is acute lymphocytic. There are an estimated 1,800 new cases each year. This type of leukemia is believed to arise most often from an abnormal lymphoid stem cell, although in a minority of cases the malignant clones are somewhat differentiated—a progeny cell population that has already begun development into B cells or T cells. Therefore, in about 75 percent of cases, the predominant abnormal cell population is extremely immature, while in the remainder of cases some markers of either B cell or T cell differentiation are present in the malignant cells.

Upon diagnosis of acute lymphocytic leukemia, the leukemic cells may or may not be significant in the blood, but will be apparent in the bone marrow and often in lymphoid organs—chiefly the spleen and lymph nodes. Some newly diagnosed patients show leukemic-cell spread to the liver, the tissues and organs in the upper torso, and the central nervous system (CNS). There is a peak incidence of acute lymphocytic leukemia between two and four years of age; a falling incidence approaching adolescence; a low rate until age sixty-five; and a slowly increasing rate thereafter.

The front-line treatment of acute lymphocytic leukemia is chemotherapy—the administration of anti-leukemia drugs, usually several different drugs in combination. Remissions—the apparent absence of leukemic cells—are attained by almost 90 percent of patients, and are usually brought about in one to two weeks of intensive treatment in the hospital. Patients continue to take maintenance drugs, at home and on periodic visits to the hospital, for a period of years (usually three to five). The maintenance drugs are often different from those administered during initial treatment, and are in lower dosages, so the patient is much less debilitated and can usually lead a fairly normal life.

The most common types of leukemia in adults are chronic lymphocytic, with some 7,600 new cases annually, and acute myelocytic, with an estimated 6,800 new cases annually.

Chronic lymphocytic leukemia is a malignancy that takes hold along the line of B cell differentiation in about 98 percent of cases (the remainder of cases involve a T cell line). In the vast majority of cases, the leukemic cell population appears to derive from a single B cell, so that all the leukemic cells are capable of producing only one specific antibody.

Because the disease progresses slowly, when there are still numbers of normal B cells present to produce a range of antibodies, and normal blood cells of other types, there may be few if any symptoms in early stages. If discovered in this relatively non-threatening stage—and it often happens accidently, when the patient has blood tests for other reasons—the leukemia may be left untreated, and the patient may live a normal life for a number of years, without any potentially debilitating therapy programs.

In later stages, there is a marked reduction in the number of normal B cells and the other varieties of blood cells, and patients may be subject to anemia and infections. When the disease becomes active, it may be treated with chemotherapy. Chronic lymphocytic leukemia has its highest incidence in elderly males, and does not occur in children.

Acute myelocytic leukemia (also known as acute granulocytic or myelogenous leukemia) is believed to originate in a stem cell committed to the myeloid line of differentiated myeloid cells. Abnormal granulocytes are common, and often red blood cells, platelets, and monocytes also are developmentally deficient and malfunctional.

When the level of primitive myeloid cells in the blood is extremely high, there is the likelihood of hemorrhage and general immobility of the white blood cells; leukemic cell invasion into tissues near the blood vessels can occur rapidly if the disease is uncontrolled. This type of leukemia has its highest incidence in those fifty-five and over, the incidence increasing with age. It can occur also in adolescents and children, at an annual rate of about ten to fifteen cases per million.

Acute myelocytic leukemia is much more difficult to control than acute lymphocytic with tolerable dosages of chemotherapy or for extended periods of time. Although remissions can now be obtained in almost 80 percent of patients, only about 20 percent of patients survive, on the average, five years or longer. Antileukemia immunizations and bone marrow transplants (see chapter 3) are two treatments being investigated that show promise in prolonging the lives of acute myelocytic leukemia patients.

Chronic myelocytic leukemia is characterized by a prominent overproduction of abnormal granulocytes or less differentiated myeloid cells, but, in contrast to the cells of acute myelocytic leukemia, the aberrant cells generally show a normal capacity for maturation. The main problem is one of cell proliferation, although the aberrant cells are often defectively functional as well. A specific identifying chromosomal defect, called the "Philadelphia chromosome," is present in affected cells of the erythrocyte, megakaryocyte, and monocyte-macrophage lines of differentiation as well. This indicates that the disease arises at the myeloid stem cell level, or perhaps even at the progenitor-pluripotent stem cell level.

Chronic myelocytic leukemia is treated with chemotherapy, and, although remissions can be obtained, they last only a few years on the average (although some patients have remained in remission for ten years and longer). The disease unfortunately usually enters an acute phase known as myeloblastic crisis, resembling acute myelocytic leukemia, and is then treated like the acute variety. It is primarily found in older adults, although it can occur in young adults and adolescents.

There is a rare form of leukemia, called erythroleukemia, in which the predominant malignant cell type, released into the blood, is an intermediate-stage stem cell that can be identified as committed to develop into a red blood cell. Although the predominant abnormal cell population consists of these primitive red blood cells, the disease also often involves the proliferation of abnormal cells all along the myeloid line of cell development, so the disease may well originate in a myeloid stem cell.

In patients with leukemias that involve abnormal cells of the myeloid line, large masses of platelets, or even megakaryocytes themselves, may appear in the blood. There is also an uncommon type of leukemia, called megakaryocytic leukemia, in which the predominant abnormal blood cell population consists of malignant megakaryocytes.

In monocytic leukemia, the predominant malignant cell population is made up of abnormal myeloid cells demonstrating certain "markers" which identify the cells as those differentiating into monocytes; the cells demonstrate phagocytic activity in the laboratory. Monocytic leukemia strikes the macrophage's precursor cells, and is often described as a leukemia affecting cells of the monocytic-macrophage line of differentiation. A less frequently used term for this category is histiocytic leukemia.

Related Diseases

Most scientists now believe that Hodgkin's disease and other malignant lymphomas (tumors of the lymphoid tissue), including multiple myeloma (primary tumor of the bone marrow), are malignancies along a continuum with the leukemias. These diseases involve primarily the lymphocytes, but differ from the leukemias in that they often form tumors (clumping of cells in particular tissues). The lymphomas are now classified in the same ways used to distinguish the leukemias: according to predominant abnormal white blood cell type, and by degree of differentiation of the transformed cell population.

Hodgkin's disease differs from other lymphomas in that it is usually localized, in early stages, to lymph nodes in one area of the lymph system. The peak concentration of the 7,400 yearly cases of Hodgkin's disease is in persons in their twenties and thirties.

Symptoms of Leukemia

The onset of leukemia can resemble cold symptoms. There may also be fatigue, paleness, loss of weight and appetite, night sweats, bone and joint pain, fever, and a recent history of repeated infections from which the individual does not appear to have completely recovered. More tangible symptoms include swelling of the gums, red skin blotches, numerous bruises, and nosebleeds or other hemorrhaging. Physician examination may reveal anemia and enlargement of the lymph nodes, spleen, and liver.

Diagnosis

The first step in diagnosis is the examination of a blood sample under the microscope. Suspicious findings include low levels of hemoglobin or a low red blood cell count; low levels of one type of white blood cell accompanied by normal or raised levels of another type; or a very high level of total white blood cells. There is likely to be a low platelet count. There also may be high levels of immature forms of one type of white blood cell found in the sample.

Infectious mononucleosis, blood derangements caused by tuberculosis bacilli, and other infections or drug-induced blood changes can produce a blood-sample profile that mimics acute leukemia. These conditions can generate an increase in the number of white blood cells in the blood, including immature forms. These, however, are reversible or self-limiting conditions, which are readily indicated by laboratory tests that can induce these benign immature cells to differentiate and mature.

Diagnosis of leukemia must be established by the microscopic examination of a sample of bone marrow tissue. Normal bone marrow appears in Figure 3A. Following local anesthetic, bone marrow specimens are drawn by needle biopsy, usually from the breastbone or the bone at the top of the hip. The specimen will reveal any accumulation of white blood cells, whether they appear monotonous (clonal) or varied, and whether the proliferation and crowding (if present) has obliterated normal structures of the

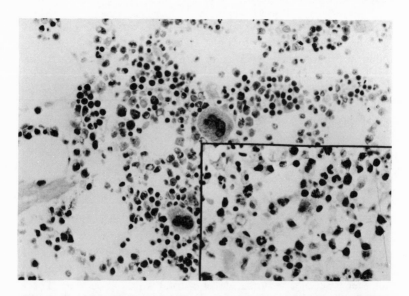

Figure 3a. Magnified photo of a normal bone marrow sample. The areas that appear empty are accumulations of fat, normally the major constituent of marrow. The cells include the various stem cells or precursor cells that differentiate into red cells (those with a dark or dense aspect), white cells (those larger cells that appear lighter and granular), and the very large cells, called megakaryocytes, that produce the platelets. Normal bone marrow shows a variety of blood-forming cells in different stages of maturation. The photo inset shows some of these cells in greater detail, at a higher magnification. *(Andrew G. Huvos, M.D.)*

marrow. Leukemic bone marrow appears in Figure 3B. An estimate of the relative proportions of the various normal blood cell populations also can be made.

Under the electron microscope, structural differences between leukemic cells and normal stem cells, immature cells, or only slightly differentiated cells may be apparent. Leukemic cells often show a disparity in age between nucleus and cytoplasm (the "factory" of the cell between the nucleus and the outer surface): the nucleus has earmarks of a young, dividing cell, while the cytoplasm is that of a more mature cell. The nucleus is usually larger than normal and often has much more DNA—the molecules of genetic material.

Various other laboratory tests will distinguish leukemic cells from normal primitive blood cells, including analysis of their products and their responses to substances that are known to specifically stimulate or inhibit normal cells. The overabundant

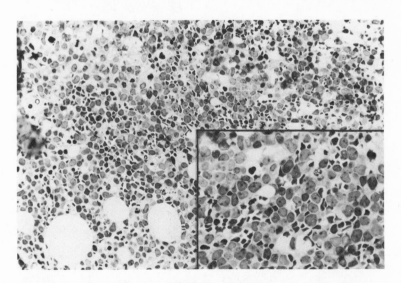

Figure 3b. Magnified photo of a bone marrow sample showing untreated acute leukemia. The normal variety of blood-forming cells has been lost, and largely replaced by leukemic white cell precursors; these have also infiltrated the fatty marrow. The photo inset shows some of these leukemic cells in greater detail, at a higher magnification. *(Andrew G. Huvos, M.D.)*

white cell type, if it is determined that the cells are leukemic, will be classified as described earlier, according to lineage (myeloid or lymphoid) and developmental stage. In order to determine the best approach to treatment, it is essential to distinguish the type and "species" of leukemic cell.

CHAPTER TWO

CAUSES, COINCIDENCES, AND RISK FACTORS IN THE GENESIS OF LEUKEMIA

It is estimated by scientists that the average individual may harbor between 100 and 1,000 malignant cells on any given day. Normally, these affected cells will repair their damage, die, or be inactivated or destroyed by the immune-response system.

Current statistics predict that one out of every four Americans will develop some type of cancer. Cancer is predominantly a disease of middle and old age, and persons near age seventy account for a higher number of cases than those in any other age group. Even though we may not know the exact mechanisms of cancer development, it nonetheless makes more sense to us that cancer might arise in the elderly, due to cumulative and damaging exposures, and deterioration of function and resistance. We are horrified when children are stricken with cancer, and our reasoning regarding cancer in the elderly (or high-risk groups such as smokers or asbestos workers) doesn't hold up.

This chapter will deal with the current findings and theories regarding conducive settings for the genesis of cancer—and leukemia in particular; likely causes and contributing factors; and some indicators of susceptibility to malignancies.

Leukemic cells, and malignant cells in general, are transformed cells. They are different from normal cells in ways that scientists are still cataloguing, ways that involve changed structural and functional properties. Every malignant cell has lost, to some degree, control over its schedule of progress or performance; but usually this is betrayed in the workings or appearance of its surface structures—deviances that will usually summon an immune response and destruction. A significant property of malignant cells, as opposed to temporarily malfunctioning cells that can repair and restore themselves, is that they have accepted, and perpetuate, their deviant orders and activities.

In some persons, the transformation of a normal cell into a leukemic cell is subtle enough, or confusing or overwhelming enough, to manipulate the cell into complicity with a chromosomal or functional deviance and/or an attacker. The cell "blindly" follows its new orders, including the order to multiply. In those persons who develop a malignancy of threatening proportions, this cellular complicity and proliferation somehow evade the alarm systems of the immune response.

The direct cause or causes of leukemia in humans remains unknown. Scientists believe that the causes involve a complex interaction of individual genetic and biochemical factors; the possible participation of a virus or a virus-like alteration of the genetic script; and environmental factors, including exposure to certain carcinogens or radiation. The individual's immune-response system plays a vital role in both resistance to leukemia and development of the disease.

GENES, GENETIC DEFECTS, AND DAMAGE

In every normal person, each cell—except sperm and egg cells—has forty-six chromosomes, threads of genetic information appearing as twenty-two matched pairs plus two sex chromosomes. The chromosomes consolidate and line up in the nucleus of the cell at the time of cell division.

When the cell divides, the chromosomes copy themselves (a process known as replication), and then move apart as the parent cell pinches itself in half—trapping one complete set of chromosomes in each of the two daughter cells. When the cell is resting or too mature for reproduction, the chromosomal material also relaxes into seeming disarray. In an adult human, at least 4 million cells are dividing every second.

In each cell, strung out like beads along the chromosome threads, are over 100,000 gene units, each one located in a definite position on a particular chromosome. Genes are composed of double strands of DNA (deoxyribonucleic acid), molecues arranged in a series of four chemical subunits called nucleotides. DNA was discovered in 1868, but was considered to be a simple, even prosaic molecule. Not until 1953 was the structure of the "double helix," the interwoven DNA strands, elucidated. DNA resembles a twisted ladder, with the rungs representing the chemical bonds between each strand. The long strands of DNA are in fact the repository of the genes, an organism's "master blueprint" of heredity (see Figure 4).

DNA relates the chemical messages that tell every cell what it can do and what its daughter cells can become. The order in which the subunits or nucleotides are arranged along the double strands of DNA directs the construction of an entire organism—whether bacterium, mouse, or human being. Duplicating itself is a vital task for DNA in cells that must rapidly proliferate in order to meet the demands of a growing organism; for example, a fertilized human egg cell (genetically complete with twenty-three chromosomes

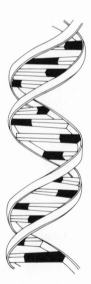

Figure 4. Diagrammatic representation of the spiral, double-stranded DNA molecule. The *sequence* of the chemical subunits (the paired "rungs" in the drawing) along the twisted strands encodes the genetic information. *(Paul Zuckerman)*

furnished by the egg cell and twenty-three donated by the sperm cell) yields, within nine months, a fetus composed of some 6,000 billion cells. DNA must be doubled before a cell can divide.

The separate DNA contributions of each parent (the sperm cell and the egg cell) account for variation as well as continuity among generations of individuals. This fixed allotment of DNA assures the same "genetic dowry" to all the cells of a given individual. DNA provides for this legacy of traits and potential by encoding plans for the cell's most distinguishing and important products—proteins, which are of many types and have widely varying roles in the body's maintenance. Proteins are crucial to an organism's existence and are the largest component (after water) of most animal and human cells. DNA is thus the authority for many of a cell's activities. It is the cell's ability, via DNA, to build up large and complex molecules—such as proteins—from simpler components that distinguishes biological systems from inorganic systems such as crystals.

DNA remains within the cell's command post, the nucleus. The cell's system for recognizing which genes (DNA segments that encode plans for a given protein) should be paid attention to at any given moment is not known. However, it is known that in order to effect a given gene's instructions for protein assembly, interpreters and executors are needed. These are the roles of the molecules of RNA (ribonucleic acid), a close chemical cousin to DNA that is single-stranded.

With the aid of enzymes, a single strand of RNA is constructed that corresponds exactly to a particular strand of DNA that is giving orders at the moment. The strand of RNA is formed in the nucleus, then moves out into the cell's cytoplasm, its chemical factory. Here the RNA serves as the medium and the message: using the information derived from DNA, RNA orders the assembly (again with the aid of enzymes) of the requisite chemicals, known as amino acids, for the building of the ordered protein. The resultant protein is then put to work; its job may keep it with the issuing cell, or it may be sent out for duties elsewhere.

There are twenty common amino acids—several of them essential in human nutrition. They can be assembled in variously ordered strings (depending on the particular activated gene's instructions); and the length and sequencing of the amino acids determines the character of each protein. An average protein usually has several hundred linked amino acids.

DNA is not autonomous in guiding a cell's activities. Influential and sometimes decisive contributions to a cell's priorities and agenda can be made by chemical messages (e.g., hormones) received from other cells, or from outside sources (e.g., foreign organic substances). Limitations are even imposed by a cell's stores at any given moment, such as its supply of free nucleotides, calcium, and certain phosphates which are an important energy source.

The genes' instigation of construction—primarily, of proteins—is their best-known role; but the important functions of DNA segments known as regulatory genes are being revealed in genetics research. These studies are just beginning but it appears that the capabilities of regulatory genes range from issuing "start" and "stop" orders for the transcription, by RNA, of a particular gene's code into a desired protein, to being "master switches" that can trigger a cell into division or dormancy, or can activate whole blocks of genes.

In addition, there are long, repetitive sequences of DNA scattered along the chromosomes in hundreds of thousands of copies whose function, if any, is not understood. Unlike other DNA, they do not carry instructions for making proteins. They may serve a back-up or "fail-safe" function—although many scientists do not believe DNA anticipates a possible need for spare parts; or these DNA sequences may be simply silent, evolutionary baggage—what some investigators have dubbed "selfish DNA"—that simply replicates itself and is of no use to the host (see Figure 5).

Each of the billions of body cells (except sperm and egg cells, which contain only half the genetic complement) contains, as far as is presently known, exactly the same genetic material—the same allotment of DNA. How, then, do cells develop specificity? In other words, how do some cells become blood cells, and others lung, skin, brain, or bone cells? The key to this is the process called cell differentiation, which starts during the formation of the human embryo.

In the cells of each type of developing tissue, only the genes that keep those cells alive and are related to its specialized functions are used, or expressed. The rest of the genes—the vast

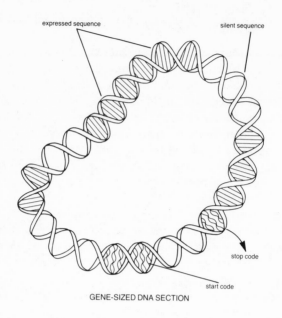

expressed sequence   silent sequence

stop code

start code

GENE-SIZED DNA SECTION

Figure 5. Diagram of DNA segment, showing expressed, regulatory, and silent (nonexpressed) sequences. Even in the DNA segment of a small gene that encodes a "short" protein, there may be sequences that are not transcribed into RNA (or are dropped when the RNA oversees protein production). These nontranscribed sequences may serve a regulatory function ("start" and "stop" codes); and may include silent sequences that could serve as a contingency reserve, or may be simply DNA evolutionary baggage. *(Harvey Offenhartz, Inc.)*

majority of them—are normally permanently "turned off," that is, superseded or overridden in an orderly way. The set of genes expressed in lung cells, for example, would be different from those working in brain cells. Among the significant characteristics of cells that have been malignantly transformed are anachronistic proteins—gene products that would only be appropriate in fetal cells; or the expression of genes (recognized by the proteins they successfully order) in the wrong type of cell (e.g., a blood cell producing quantities of an enzyme that is normally restricted to skin cells).

It is only with the remarkable advances in molecular biology that began in the 1970s that scientists are now able to examine genes directly. Techniques such as cell fusion and gene splicing (see chapter 5), and sophisticated instruments such as electron microscopes and DNA synthesizers, are allowing a gene's chemical message to be read. By the early 1980s, techniques were developed to unravel the *way* DNA codes for proteins, enabling scientists to read what representative gene-units are encoding, and even to manufacture workable copies of encoding DNA.

Scientists had broken the genetic code—at least for structural genes encoding proteins. They had learned that each nucleotide consists of a sugar residue, phosphate group, and a "base." The four bases are adenine (A), thymine (T), guanine (G), and cytosine (C). The bases bond to each other to form the characteristic DNA double helix; adenine always bonds to thymine, and cytosine always bonds to guanine. A linear sequence of three DNA nucleotide bases codes for one amino acid, one protein building block for the cell. For example, the sequence adenine, thymine, adenine (ATA), codes for the amino acid tyrosine; and the sequence guanine, adenine, thymine (GAT) codes for the amino acid leucine (see Figure 6).

A transcriptional dictionary has been developed that now allows scientists to decipher the possible DNA codes for all amino acids; by analyzing a given, encoding DNA segment, scientists can deduce the amino-acid formula of the gene's ordered protein. Conversely, with developing technology, scientists are able to rapidly read a given protein's amino-acid string and deduce the DNA sequences that are responsible (see Figure 7). New, automated instrumentation is reducing into days and even hours the time for completing translations that just a few years ago took months to make. The translations completed in 1981 quadrupled the total of gene-sized, DNA segments whose chemical code is known.

What has all this to do with practical medical concerns? It can lead to chromosomal "read-outs" on individuals, making it possible to trace defective genes that may be responsible for abnormal proteins that are in turn linked to serious diseases. It will allow doctors to acknowledge or rule out a genetic basis for proteins that are abnormal either in quality or quantity. The potential for another medical application lies in deciphering the DNA coding for proteins that can be medically useful. This work has already

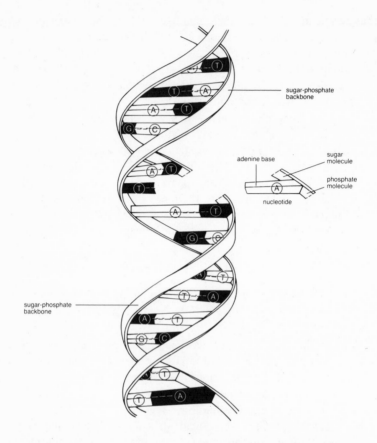

Figure 6. Diagrammatic representation of DNA, the "master blue-print" of heredity as well as the instigator of many cellular activities. The twisted strands around the outside of the DNA molecule are sugar-phosphate attachments; the inside paired bases, and their sequencing, are the essence of the genetic code. Nucleotides, which consist of one base plus its sugar-phosphate attachments, when expressed linearly and assembled in triplets, encode amino acids—the building blocks of proteins.

When DNA replicates prior to cell division, the strands unwind, and the paired nucleotide bases separate (the rungs "unzip" at the black-white juncture); each single strand with its attached chemical sequences then serves as a template for the building of new complementary strands. Thus the DNA is doubled, and each daughter molecule is an exact copy of the parent; when the cell divides, each daughter cell will have a complete array of double-stranded DNA. *(Paul Zuckerman)*

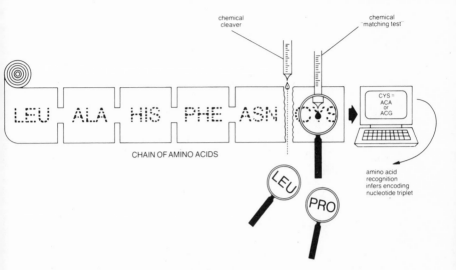

Figure 7. "Reading" proteins to trace their home base in the genes. Recognizing amino acids that make up a protein allows, with the aid of the genetic-code dictionary, inference as to the encoding DNA nucleotides. Chemical separation, and recognition processing of a protein's amino acid chain, permit reasoning backwards to possible encoding DNA sequences; thus a protein's chromosomal "home" can be located. *(Harvey Offenhartz, Inc.)*

led to the manufacture of certain synthetic hormones (e.g., human insulin, human growth hormone) that can be given to persons with deficiencies in natural production.

How does this tie in with cancer and leukemia? Pronounced and numerous changes in protein quantity or quality—often apparent in proteins found loose in the blood or imbedded on malignant cell surfaces—are associated with most, and perhaps all, types of cancer. These proteins can wreak havoc with the malignant cells' internal dynamics and priorities, as well as with their communication with other cells, including those responsible for immune surveillance. The list of proteins implicated in malignancy is presently comprised of those that can be recognized on the basis of relative scarcity or overabundance; peculiar positioning on the cell surface; incomplete or otherwise faulty structure; abnormal expression (e.g., developmental throwbacks such as fetal proteins, appearance in the wrong type of cell); and foreign origin (e.g., viruses).

It is one thing to determine abnormal proteins, and quite another to determine whether or not they are due to faulty genes— and if so, where on the chromosomes such genes are located. Although inherited, known genetic abnormalities are linked with relatively few forms of cancer, the scientific evidence increasingly implicates genetic disturbance—in structural or regulatory genes— as a necessary precondition, inherited or acquired, for the development of cancer.

Genetic Defects, Damage, and Vulnerability

Scientists have now located, or "mapped," several hundred genes, including one or more on each of the human chromosomes. One of the prime objectives of such research is to pinpoint genes linked to human hereditary disease. For example, it is now known which portion of chromosome 21 is defective in the individual with Down's syndrome, or Mongolism—even the particular chemical aberration responsible has been identified. As a result of the piece-by-piece examination of proteins that current technology permits, it can be inferred that the smallest changes in DNA coding can sometimes have powerful effects: it has been discovered that sickle-cell anemia is characterized by hemoglobin that differs from normal hemoglobin in only one out of several hundred amino acids.

Many other diseases, including a number of those that involve immune-response deficiencies, have been linked to genetic defects. Chronic myelocytic leukemia is associated with a defect called the "Philadelphia chromosome," in which a missing portion of chromosome 22 is reattached to another chromosome (see Figure 8). This genetic defect, however, may be a consequence, and not a cause, of the disease; not all patients with the disease have it, and the cell samples for those who initially do sometimes no longer show the defect when the disease is in remission.

For many people, the term genetic used to describe their condition indicates that a defect existed in the array of genes they

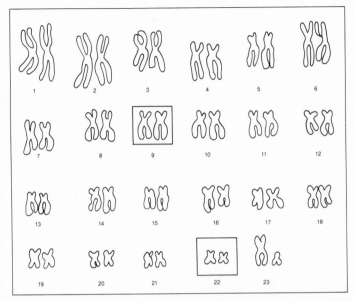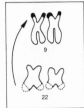

Figure 8. Diagram of a normal male's twenty-three paired chromosomes. The box on the right represents the "Philadelphia chromosome" characteristic of chronic myelocytic leukemia, in which a portion of chromosome 22 has relocated onto chromosome 9. The translocation of chromosome 22 material may also take place onto other chromosomes. *(Paul Zuckerman)*

received from their parents. It is true that we are born with our genes, and that, currently, nothing we do can improve them. (However, with the progress in gene mapping, which identifies the locations of genes responsible for various diseases, genetic repair is in the foreseeable future. Research work in this area is described in chapter 5.) But genetic errors cannot be equated with unadulterated and inevitable transmission of defects from one generation to another.

The work of the genes does not go on relentlessly, undisturbed. Far from it. Ordinary sunlight, infectious agents such as viruses, many chemicals that may be introduced into the body, and ionizing radiation (such as X-rays), are now known to be able to cause DNA damage. It was once believed that DNA was stable from generation to generation, and that if some defect or mutation (change) occurred only one of two things could happen: if the damage was severe, the cell would be killed; otherwise, the mutation would be accepted as a permanent part of the DNA.

Recent laboratory studies of cell cultures have shown that DNA damage and DNA repair probably go on constantly. In a variety of bacterial, animal, and human cells, researchers have observed that when a "mistake" inserts itself into the DNA, the marred portion is nicked and removed by two different enzymes; replaced with the right chemical combination by a third enzyme; and the repaired section is sealed into place by a fourth enzyme. This, scientists believe, is just one of the ways in which a cell repairs injury to its DNA (see Figure 9).

Errors introduced into DNA, followed by inefficient DNA repair, can lead to mutant cells. And while not all mutant cells are harmful, and many simply die, it has been shown that cells that permit mutations to stand or make clumsy efforts at repair at awkward times (e.g., during DNA replication), are often capable of becoming malignant.

A rare hereditary disease called xeroderma pigmentosum (XP), in which death from skin cancer or subsequent tumors is common, is the result of the patient's inability to repair DNA after exposure of the skin to sunlight has damaged it. It is the ultraviolet portion of sunlight that damages DNA; researchers have found, through studying skin cells in laboratory dishes, that while the cells of people without XP also can suffer DNA damage from ultraviolet light, there is a compensatory reaction initiated by the visible-light portion of sunlight, which activates cell enzymes that repair the ultraviolet-damaged DNA. (In XP patients, these compensatory enzymes are activated sluggishly, if at all.)

It has also been observed that symptoms of xeroderma pigmentosum, such as dry skin, dark-pigmented spots resembling "age spots," and progressive brain cell death mimic the changes of old age. This presents the intriguing possibility that aging, and the increased risk of malignancy that occurs with aging, may arise from cells bearing an accumulation of unrepaired errors in DNA.

Another current theory is that DNA mutations that lead to malignancy in humans do so only sometimes by virulent and preemptory dominance of a cell's life. Other times, the mutation may

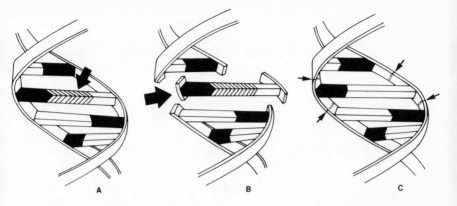

A   **B**   **C**

Figure 9a. Hatch-marked portion (arrow) of a DNA segment represents an intrusive error, which could be the result of radiation, chemical carcinogens, or virus attack, among the possible causes of DNA damage.

Figure 9b. In the normal DNA repair process, enzymes called endonucleases recognize the abnormal portion and cleave it out of the DNA strand; it will be dissolved by enzymes called exonucleases.

Figure 9c. Other enzymes, using the normal portion (black) of the damaged segment as a template, will construct a correct, complementary chemical "mate" (white); then enzymes called DNA ligases will complete the repair by sealing the renewed segment in place. *(Paul Zuckerman)*

be of a milder sort, tampering with the cell's complex code for differentiation or with regulatory genes. This theory applies to the "frozen," immature cells of the acute leukemias (preemptory takeover), and to the functionally illiterate cells seen in the chronic leukemias, which are believed to take years or even decades to develop.

A 1979 article in *The New York Times Magazine** on DNA

* Jean L. Marx, "New Clues to Cancer's Causes," 25 November 1979.

repair noted, "An error introduced into the DNA of any cell is no more likely to improve that cell than an error made by a typist who is typing *King Lear* is likely to improve Shakespeare's play." And yet some genetic mistakes are beneficial, allowing us to evolve. Mutation is surely a double-edged sword; and as the same article suggests, perhaps cancer and aging are the price we pay for the ability to evolve.

So far, only three kinds of cancer have been found to be directly associated with specific, inheritable genetic abnormalities—two types of kidney cancer, and retinoblastoma, a tumor of the eye's retina. Yet there are human families with a predisposition to a particular type of cancer, "cancer families" in which the incidence of that type of cancer is far above the norm. In one recent study* of a family that appeared predisposed to acute myelocytic leukemia (AML) through the maternal line, evidence of a defect in DNA repair has been found. The cells of at-risk relatives, when tested in laboratory cultures, were found to be easily transformed (i.e., they took on the characteristic of malignant cells) by a virus that causes leukemia in monkeys. And there are genetically determined diseases, deficiencies, and defects that are associated with a higher-than-average risk for the development of leukemia. These include Down's syndrome, two rare disorders called Bloom's syndrome and ataxia telangiectasia, certain immune-response deficiencies, and several severe anemias.

In relation to genetic changes that may occur during the lifetime of an individual, investigations have pointed to certain vulnerability indicators that are linked to susceptibility to malignancy. This work is at the experimental level, far from applicability in general screening tests, and has been done primarily on members of "cancer families."

The study of the AML family cited above showed relatives to be both lacking in capability of DNA repair and particularly vulnerable to viruses that induce animal leukemias. Other studies involve exposing cell samples from target subjects to low levels of ionizing radiation and various carcinogenic, or cancer-causing,

* "Family History Information Enables Physicians to Recognize Genetically 'At-Risk' Patients," *Journal of the American Medical Association*, 4 January 1980, vol. 243, p. 19.

chemicals. Persons whose cells are unusually vulnerable to damage from these exposures, or whose DNA shows mutation, are identified as being at increased risk for malignancy. The accuracy of the predictions based on these studies will depend on the occurrence or nonoccurrence of malignancy in the follow-up of these "tagged" individuals.

The body's handling of toxic substances forms the basis for another avenue of investigation into susceptibility to malignancy. For example, certain ingredients of tobacco smoke are proven carcinogens; it is estimated that of 1,000 people who smoke a pack of cigarettes a day for thirty years, 20 percent will probably get lung cancer.

What distinguishes that 20 percent? Research has shown that a *potentially* carcinogenic substance must change chemically, via processing steps *particular to an individual's metabolism*, into a form capable of binding to DNA or RNA and thereby causing cell mutation, to become *actually* carcinogenic. In cell studies tracing the outcome of one carcinogenic tobacco-smoke substance, researchers have discovered that four different groups of cell enzymes are involved in the effort to dispose of this foreign chemical via metabolic transformation. Their efforts will lead to the emergence of an end product that has shown up in over forty different variations of the original substance, depending on individual metabolic-pathway preferences. One particular end product of the tobacco-smoke substance has been found to be several thousand times more potent that the others, in terms of binding to DNA and causing mutation. Since researchers now know its processing steps, this knowledge may make it possible to test smokers by charting enzymatic action in cell samples that have been deliberately exposed to doses of the tobacco carcinogen. Such tests would show whether the individual's cells would transform the carcinogen into a harmless excretable substance or into the potent form that binds to DNA and causes mutation.

Most human malignancies occur in both heritable and nonheritable forms. The consensus in medical science today is that genetic defect or vulnerability to mutation is not the sole cause of malignancy, but a potential accomplice, requiring other partners to perpetuate malignant development in an individual.

Does a carcinogen cause a change in genetic information, a

mutation that can overload the DNA repair machinery if exposure to the carcinogen persists or occurs in an overwhelmingly large dosage? It appears that this situation can lead to malignant cells in some cases. Is the cancer-causing genetic information already in the cell, and does the carcinogen simply aid and abet it into taking over? It is believed by many scientists that genetic aberrations, both those inherited and those acquired (e.g., cellular invasion by microorganisms, cellular damage by carcinogens such as radiation and chemicals), generate cellular diversity, thereby setting the stage for the emergence of cell clones that have the particular abnormalities identified with cancer.

If the genes already carry the information that can lead to malignancy, where did this genetic information come from? The most recent scientific evidence persuades many researchers that viruses provide the clue to the answer.

VIRUSES AND CANCER-CAUSING GENES

Viruses are tiny infectious agents that can prey on plants and even fungi and bacteria, as well as on animals, including humans. They cannot independently sustain themselves biologically, and can reproduce only with the help of living host cells. They are definitive parasites. One of the smallest and simplest of all known viruses has only three genes, as compared with the average bacterium, which contains about 5,000 genes.

All types of viruses are simply packets of genetic material— either DNA or RNA segments, but never both—wrapped in protein coats. They also are characterized by protruding proteins— antenna-like spikes which stick onto a cell the virus plans to enter.

In a successful virus attack, the spike penetration causes the cell to engulf the whole virus; the virus heads for the cell's nucleus (often shedding coat proteins along the way), where the virus's DNA or RNA snippet is accepted as part of the cell's genetic array, and the cell is induced to make viral proteins specified by the viral genes. The final victory, however, usually goes to the host organism, if not the individual invaded cells (which may die from this "moonlighting" at the expense of their own duties). The host will mount a counterattack, including an immune response against virus particles or cells exhibiting viral proteins (an attack that includes the production of interferon—see chapter 5).

The important question here, however, is if and how certain viruses cause or contribute to the development of cancer.

Cancer-Causing Viral Mutations in Animals

Leukemia occurs throughout the vertebrate animal kingdom, and has even been found in some invertebrates. Many other types of malignancy occur in animals. It has been known for over seventy years, since the discovery of a virus that caused cancer in chickens, that viruses can induce cancer in animals. It has recently been demonstrated that transmissible viruses are strongly implicated in the majority of malignant tumors in animals, and in animal leukemia.

There were obstacles that prevented many scientists in the 1950s from readily accepting the theory that transmissible viruses were a causative agent in animal malignancies:

1. While certain virus-caused human diseases, such as polio, measles, and flu, are contagious, human cancer is not.
2. A few animal malignancies (including leukemia in chickens) appeared contagious, and could be presumably traced to a submicroscopic agent, probably a virus; however, a malignancy could arise in one offspring of a protected, laboratory-animal family in which neither parent nor any littermates had or developed cancer.
3. Tumors could be induced in animals (and in man) by a variety of chemical carcinogens or radiation.

It has since been confirmed in animal studies that certain viruses, termed oncogenic, or tumor-producing, have the ability not only to cause infection, to use the host cell's nutrients and synthesizing machinery, and to cause cell destruction; but to integrate—to chemically splice—their own genetic material into the DNA of the cells of the host animal. The case of the RNA tumor viruses overturned one of the basic tenets of biology, which was that DNA could order the production of RNA, but not the other way around. It was found in 1970 that RNA tumor viruses come equipped with an enzyme that enables the viral RNA to use *itself* as the blueprint and direct the enzyme to fashion its likeness into a strand of DNA. True to form, the DNA strand then reproduced itself to become a double strand, which could be accepted by the host cell's chromosome family (see Figure 10). For the DNA tumor viruses, the process is simpler—they just have to force their genes into the cell's DNA.

The invaded cell is now a mutant, and if the DNA repair service doesn't eject the foreign viral DNA, and the immune-response system doesn't destroy the host cell, and the cell doesn't die, the cell now has an altered but heritable blueprint for transmission to daughter cells—one that includes viral genes. In answer to the first two questions originally raised about viral responsibility for spreading a cancer, it can now be seen that the transmission is not necessarily "horizontal"—spread by contagion or contact, but can be "vertical"—genetically encoded and passed on in active or latent form, from parent to embryo (through stray mutant cells or mutant sperm or egg cells), from one generation to another. RNA tumor viruses can also induce leukemias that are horizontally transmitted—that is, promoted by contagion—in certain susceptible animals. Healthy cats exposed to leukemic cats are estimated to be 100 times more likely to develop leukemia than they otherwise would.

The third objection, the proven role of radiation and other carcinogens in the induction of animal malignancies, was countered over the years by investigations culminating in the two-step theory of cancer, now generally accepted. This theory will be discussed later in this chapter; but essentially it proposes that an underlying, cancer-conducive situation must usually pre-exist in the creature that develops cancer, but that it is contained or "on hold" until later biochemical events or assaults push the hapless cell or cells into mechanical, malignant behavior. Tumor-capable, viral genes, when integrated into a host cell, certainly can create a conducive situation; and viral genes and their products have in fact been recovered from many test animals whose cancer seemed induced by

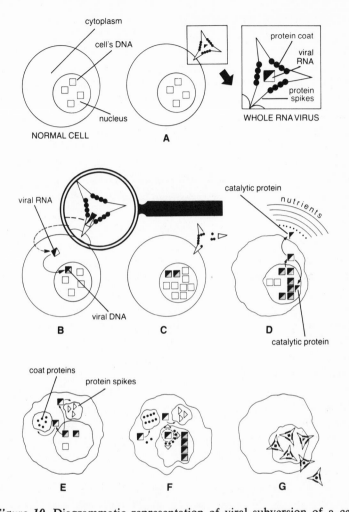

Figure 10. Diagrammatic representation of viral subversion of a cell. A normal cell is attacked by an RNA virus (A). In drawing B, the virus (magnified) inserts its genetic material—RNA—into the cell's cytoplasm; the viral RNA then moves into the cell's nucleus to direct formation of viral DNA. Most of the virus's protein coat and spikes are left behind. The viral DNA is replicated along with the cell's DNA (C). In drawing D, some viral DNA is transcribed into RNA that orders production of catalytic proteins, which stimulate the cell to take in nutrients and to replicate more viral DNA. Other viral DNA (E) is transcribed into RNA that orders production of viral protein coats and protein spikes. In drawing F, the virus begins to reassemble itself; almost all genetic activity in the cell is now devoted to virus assembly. In this hypothetical outcome, the virus dominates the cell (G), kills it, then moves on. *(Harvey Offenhartz, Inc.)*

low doses of radiation or chemical carcinogens. When a second healthy animal is inoculated with the recovered viral genes in large dosages, it too can develop cancer. Although this method is cancer-causation by onslaught, and does not fit the more usual two-step theory of cancer, it does prove that viral genes can cause cancer.

Exactly how do these mutations lead to cancer? Although all the answers are not known, and there are probably multiple routes to malignancy among individuals, much has been learned about cancer causation, and the development of leukemia in particular, by studies of RNA tumor viruses in animals, and studies of the ways viruses invade bacteria—ways that can be quite easily observed or measured.

It is important to stress at this point that RNA tumor viruses do not seem to be a major cause of human cancer. Although it is unthinkable to test human susceptibility by inoculating people with malignant animal cells, it has been demonstrated in animal tests that inoculations prepared from tumor cells of one species only occasionally cause malignancy in another species. And extracts of human tumors do not transmit malignancy when inoculated into animals.

Since viruses have evolved for survival, like other living creatures (or quasi-living, in the case of such parasites), it is reasonable to assume they would not predominantly follow a "scorched-earth" policy—or we would not be here and they would not be here. It is believed that most types of RNA tumor viruses probably represent a very old, latent infection that has been transmitted from one generation to another for many centuries. These viruses are usually silent, and, says renowned virologist and cancer researcher Ludwik Gross, M.D., "frugal and moderate in their requirements."* They have remained, says Dr. Gross, in most instances submerged, "except that an occasional cancer or leukemia develops in one of their carrier hosts.

"However, when triggered by a variety of metabolic, hormonal or chemical factors or by ionizing radiation, they become patho-

* Ludwik Gross, "Cancer and Slow Virus Diseases—Some Common Features," *The New England Journal of Medicine,* 23 August 1979, vol. 301, pp. 432–33. Reprinted by permission.

genic and cause the development of malignant tumors or leukemia in their hosts."

The class of RNA tumor viruses with which scientists are most familiar, and which Dr. Gross describes as "moderate," can often coexist fairly peaceably with the host cell, even in a new, rather than a passed-down, infection. The cell may be overworked but often suffers no damage, even when virus particles are being manufactured, and new viruses assemble and leave the cell. As noted, the viral genes are often silent, probably repressed by nearby cellular regulatory genes or policing proteins (such proteins in bacteria are known to literally sit on viral genes).

Viral genes can be triggered into activity, as Dr. Gross and others note, by a variety of internal or external factors; but new evidence indicates that the lifting of their repression is only part of the reason as to why they can cause cancer. After all, their "freedom of expression" should produce only an active viral infection. A number of investigators believe that the *positioning* of the viral genetic insertion in the host cell's DNA is critical as to its possible influence—and whether or not there will be a malignant outcome. If the insertion cripples an important regulatory gene or is near a host gene involved in cell growth—normally suppressed—a chain reaction can take place. The viral genes plus the growth-stimulating host gene take over the cell. A second, chance mutation then makes chaos of the cell's regulatory system causing cell proliferation at the expense of all else.

It is known from animal and cell studies that one gene, making one protein, can transform a cell into a malignant one, overwhelming the cell with signals to multiply. The cell becomes unable to differentiate or age.

There is another class of RNA tumor viruses whose workings have been unraveled only in the past few years; the viruses are much more virulent in inducing malignancies, and a number of them have been studied in detail in relation to their ability to cause leukemia and related malignancies such as sarcomas (cancers of bone and connective tissue). These RNA viruses possess an *additional gene* to the usual viral genetic packets that are devoted to the construction of the virus and its integration into a host cell. The extra gene has been termed an *oncogene*, because it and its singular protein product, an enzyme (of a family called kinases, which are involved in energy transfers), have been found to be capable of solely causing malignant transformation of normal cells in laboratory cultures.

The action of these viral oncogenes (found, so far, in chickens, mice, rats, cats, and monkeys) appears to take precedence over all other genes in an invaded cell, and to cause overt leukemia in its animal victims within days or weeks, in contrast to the many months required for disease manifestation induced by the "moderate" RNA tumor viruses. Studies indicate that the oncogene must be continuously expressed to maintain the cancer cell as a cancer cell. It does this through its enzyme product, which, although not yet well understood by scientists, is known to be involved in energy transactions in the cell that convince the cell it is a young and growing newcomer and must devote itself exclusively to division. The enzyme acts like a perverse fountain of youth, bestowing indefinite infancy or adolescence on captive cells —at the expense of life-sustaining functions in the host organism.

Natural "Cancer-Genes" in Animals and Humans

Cancer researchers specializing in virology have been hot on the trail of RNA tumor viruses for decades; and the discovery of specific oncogenes in some of them cleared up the confusion as to moderate (RNA tumor viruses without an oncogene) versus virulent (viruses with an oncogene) induction of cancer in the animal victims. These researchers discovered virus-like particles— that is, genetic snippets resembling viral oncogenes—that began consistently turning up in the DNA of normal animal cells as well as malignant cells (located using radioactive oncogenes that would bind to these presumably normal "twin" genes and illuminate them).

Pursuing the oncogenes in normal animal cells, researchers made a startling discovery: The widely dispersed oncogenes turned out to be "extra" genes indeed—genes that were not native to the viruses. Says cancer virologist J. Michael Bishop of the University of California at San Francisco, in a recent article in *Scientific*

American:* "It has turned out that the genes are not even peculiar to cancer cells. They are present and functioning in normal cells as well, and they may be as necessary for the life of the normal cell as they appear to be for the unrestrained growth of a cancer. A final common pathway by which all tumors arise may be part of the genetic dowry of every living cell."

A coincidental finding that bolstered this research was that viruses tend to make off with gene segments from the DNA of cells that they have invaded. When they invade their next cell (or when their descendants invade another individual) and splice their genetic packet into the cell's DNA, the genetic donation may be part native-virus DNA and part DNA literally "ripped off" from previous host cells. The normal cellular "cancer gene" is slightly different from the viral oncogene—in ways that are typical of differences in genetic coding between viruses and higher organisms: the viral gene is streamlined, while the cellular gene is piecemeal, divided here and there by segments that do not show up in the ordering of the protein product. These DNA "spacers" may serve a regulatory purpose in the host DNA; but the virus, when it appropriates the animal gene, discards all DNA that is not strictly useful.

The enzymes produced by the various RNA virus oncogenes so far studied, and by the nearly identical "cancer genes" in normal animals, are, as may be expected, very similar. The enzymes, whose functions have as yet only been glimpsed by investigators, seem to stimulate preparations for cell reproduction, and the site of action seems to be the cell membrane. Some sixteen different RNA virus oncogenes *having normal cellular counterparts* have been discovered as of mid-1983, all related to leukemia and sarcoma. The discovery of leukemia-capable normal genes was an accidental offshoot of finding the model "extra" genes in viruses that could cause rapid leukemia. Many investigators now believe that a variety of other cellular "cancer genes" exist and can be activated to cause the different types of cancer—even though viruses may not be so serendipitously involved as pathfinders.

* J. Michael Bishop, "Oncogenes," *Scientific American,* March 1982, vol. 246, pp. 80–92.

The study of viral oncogenes has pointed the way to an observable mechanism of cancer induction; and much of this work has involved oncogenes that cause leukemia in animals. Dr. David Baltimore, Nobel-Prize-winning biologist at the Massachusetts Institute of Technology, is making an intensive study of an RNA viral oncogene that causes leukemia in mice; and his preliminary findings indicate that the transport functions performed by the oncogene's ordered enzyme rob key energy chemicals from the cell and pass them on to favored proteins at the cell's surface—probably the enzymes themselves.* This would serve as a continuous self-stimulation. The enzyme may also induce leukemia by continually importing molecules that keep the cell growing (i.e., aim it toward division), or by acting as a receptor for hormones or hormone-like substances that are given preferential binding privileges and that stimulate cell reproduction.

Using a fluorescent antibody that specifically binds to the oncogene's enzyme, Dr. Baltimore searched normal mouse cells for a counterpart enzyme: he found the enzyme predominantly in normal T lymphocytes and their precursors. However, in mice infected with the viral oncogene, the leukemic cells are B lymphocytes, and the enzyme is produced in amounts 100 times greater than normal. Dr. Baltimore suggests that the viral oncogene causes leukemia by producing too much of a normal cell product or by producing it in cells of a type not equipped to handle it.

The viral-oncogene theory of leukemia causation in animals adapted to leukemia induction by alternative routes would propose that a natural "leukemia gene" could be "turned on" by any nearby DNA damage that by itself, or through the attraction of overzealous DNA repair enzymes, liberates the gene for expression. Another theory is that viral DNA segments that normally flank virus genes and order their frenetic activity might attach themselves to the natural "leukemia gene" and command it to overproduce (this has been done with normal cells in the laboratory). It has been observed that an RNA tumor virus *without an oncogene* that causes lymphoma in chickens *is almost always* inserted

---

* Quoted in "Unifying Genetic Theme for RNA Viral Cancer?", *Medical Tribune,* 28 November 1979, p. 10.

in the immediate vicinity of a recognized natural "cancer gene," and that the expression of the cellular gene is greatly amplified.

The above discoveries relating to viral oncogenes and normal, counterpart "cancer genes" that are "not alien intruders but normal, indeed essential, genes run amok," in the words of Dr. Bishop, have just been made over the past few years. In summary, the evidence to date indicates the following:

1. Viruses bearing oncogenes, believed stolen from animal hosts where they served a natural, growth-related purpose, infect another animal host where the gene is integrated and expressed. The gene must be liberated from cellular controls, and the new host's immune system must fail to check the invaded cell; then the cell and its new stimulant-trafficking enzyme become the purveyors of a clone of malignantly transformed cells.

2. Animals and humans possess natural "leukemia genes," believed to be the origin of viral oncogenes, stolen from animals by RNA viruses in the fairly recent past; in the rightful owner these genes are responsible for a growth-related enzyme that is produced only in certain cells or at certain times, or in other cells in very small amounts. But if the natural "leukemia gene" is freed of normal restraints, as by a DNA mutation that "turns it on," its enzyme product can dominate the cell and freeze it in a state of perpetual division, transforming it into a leukemic cell.

3. Although most of this investigative work has been done with viral oncogenes and their prototype, natural "leukemia genes" that can cause leukemia or sarcoma in animals (or leukemic changes in cells in the laboratory), many investigators believe that other types of cancer can be traced to other—as yet undiscovered—natural "cancer genes" in the body.

4. It is yet unproven that normal "leukemia genes" can be "turned on" in a healthy animal without some

participation by an RNA tumor virus—either past (latent viral genes with or without a specific onco-gene) or present (active RNA virus infection). Although it seems highly probable that other causes of DNA mutation (e.g., carcinogens, radiation) might free a natural "cancer gene" and transform the cell into a malignant one, so far this has been accomplished in the laboratory only with some form of virus participation, such as the insertion into normal cells of viral-regulatory or flanking DNA segments, which order any adjacent gene to work harder than usual.

A Direct Virus Role in Human Leukemia?

Viruses are known to be quite species-specific; that is, certain types of viruses can survive only within a particular plant or animal host-species. If viral genetic material has been integrated into the genes of a particular family line within a species, descendants of that line have an inborn genetic mutation that may carry a high risk of later cancer. And some family lines carry genetic "processing" peculiarities that make them highly suscepti-ble to cell mutations, including viral integration.

RNA tumor viruses that can induce leukemia and other cancers in animals are considered minimally infectious, under normal con-ditions, in humans. Yet for decades many virologists have be-lieved, but have not been able to prove, that viruses must influence human cancer as they have been proven to do in animal cancer.

Evidence for a viral role in human cancer is circumstantial, but certainly exists. RNA viruses have been implicated particularly in acute myelocytic leukemia and breast cancer in humans. The enzyme that allows RNA viruses to transcribe their genetic packet into host-acceptable DNA—an enzyme believed to be exclusive to this family of viruses—has been found in virtually every sample of fresh, human acute leukemia cells.

An additional note about nonhuman animal leukemia: the cross-species capability of viruses has been demonstrated in studies of leukemia in the gibbon ape. In 1973 an RNA virus was isolated from an ape that had acute myelocytic leukemia; and when the virus was inoculated into a healthy ape, that animal too developed leukemia. It is also believed that leukemia in apes arose in the mid-1800s, and that the responsible virus is a predator that previously ranged only among mice.

An investigation reported early in 1982* strengthened the possibilities of a viral role in at least one type of human leukemia. Reported by a team of researchers from the National Cancer Institute (NCI) and three universities in Japan, the study of six Japanese patients with T cell leukemia turned up antibodies in their blood samples against a type of RNA virus. T cell leukemia accounts for less than 1 percent of all leukemia cases in the United States, but has an unusually high incidence in the islands of southwestern Japan. Blood samples of randomly selected healthy persons from that area did not contain the antibodies. NCI spokesmen say the virus may serve as a promotional agent for leukemia in persons who are genetically susceptible or who are exposed to unknown carcinogens in the environment.

Linked to human malignancies by more direct evidence than the RNA viruses are the family of DNA viruses known as herpes viruses (of which more than seventy varieties are known, most of which attack only animals). Until relatively recently, types of herpes viruses that attack humans—and only five types are known to do so—were considered to cause mild (cold sores) or even serious (venereal disease) conditions, but were not suspected to have life-threatening potential. It is estimated that almost 95 percent of adult Americans harbor latent herpes viruses of some type; they are spread by person-to-person contact. They are sturdily constructed, and about four times the size of the average flu virus.

During the past twenty-five years, extensive study has been done on a herpes virus known as the Epstein-Barr virus (EBV). It was firmly established in 1969 that EBV causes infectious mononucleosis, the debilitating illness that appears to strike primarily adolescents and young adults. EBV specifically attaches to B lymphocytes, and stimulates them to divide; this triggers a special "suppressor" population among T lymphocytes to inhibit the pro-

* "New Data Suggest Virus May Cause Form of Human Cancer," *The New York Times*, 12 February 1982.

liferation, and some of them kill outright the virus-bearing cells. In infectious mononucleosis, there is an intense cellular action and reaction, but normally the disease subsides; it is self-limiting.

Scientists are almost certain that EBV is causally linked to a malignancy fairly common among children in certain sections of Africa, a disease called Burkitt's lymphoma. EBV is also considered highly suspect in its association with a malignancy of the nose and throat in the Orient. In the laboratory, EBV can transform normal primate and human cells into malignant ones. These cultured cells, when injected into animals whose immune system has been suppressed by radiation, have the potential to produce lethal tumors.

What has been shown is that EBV can serve as a co-conspirator in the development of malignant cells. It is believed that a conducive situation or prompting event is usually needed for actual malignant proliferation of cells to occur. The conducive situation could be a genetic susceptibility, such as a defect passed through the maternal line that has been found in certain cases of fatal infectious mononucleosis; and a prompting event could be another infection which overburdens the immune system—and malaria is strongly indicated in Burkitt's lymphoma.

Other herpes virus infections that are linked to human cancer include the venereal herpes simplex, believed to be a contributing factor in at least some cases of cancer of the cervix; and the hepatitis B virus, infection by which seems to precede most cases of liver cancer.

It is not known how DNA viruses such as the herpes viruses contrive their latency state, although the herpes simplex virus is known to hide out in nerve cells, erupting into reactivated infections upon various provocations ranging from a lowered immune response to stress. When the virus is active and ordering host cells to produce more viruses, the host cell will die, and the viruses will burrow into nearby cells where they can repeat the process. Certain DNA viruses that cause cancer in animals, like RNA tumor viruses, succeed in integrating their genetic packet into the DNA of host cells. However, unlike RNA viruses, the DNA tumor viruses must remain quiet—not producing new infectious virus—in the genes, although they may express bits of viral information; if they start producing viral progeny, the host cell will die.

At least four different families of DNA viruses are linked to malignancies in animals, including several types of herpes viruses that induce leukemia in certain primates. It is not yet known whether any DNA viruses carry oncogenes, matched by prototype, natural "cancer genes" in normal cells.

Recent evidence indicates that most viruses linked to cancer causation act in a generic way as mutation agents, similar to other agents or factors that may (1) predispose the host to develop a malignancy or (2) serve as the prompting event in the actual development of a malignancy. Other times, according to the work described in this section, the virus may carry an animal gene or zero in on a similar gene in its victim that, if "turned on" in the host, can overwhelm the cell with commands to multiply, and lead to an expanding clone of malignantly transformed cells.

SELF-DEFENSE AND THE IMMUNE-RESPONSE SYSTEM

The body as a rule is ruthless about its autonomy and its protocol for guests, and can be insatiable in its quest against intruders. Dr. Lewis Thomas, chancellor at New York City's Memorial Sloan-Kettering Cancer Center, speculates that this capacity first evolved from primordial sensing mechanisms needed by simple life forms to search out others mutually dependent for survival; and that it then became insistent and formalized, developing into the "wisdom" needed to keep symbiosis and merging from getting out of hand.*

It is true also that we have, over our long evolution, made exceptions to our boundary rules, and still allow certain peaceful coexistences. Dr. Thomas asserts that an integral part of human cells called the mitochrondria, now a fixture in processing food energy, is an ancient borrowing from bacteria. We know about the harmless and permitted nesting of bacteria in various parts of the human body, such as the gastrointestinal system. And we are aware of the mutations, the conditionings, and other mistakes—

* Lewis Thomas, *The Lives of a Cell* (New York: The Viking Press, 1974), pp. 1–29.

such as the incorporation of viral coding into our genes—that may not harm us. Mutations, some of which may allow us to evolve, may be passed from generation to generation.

In general, however, the body's tough obstacle course, its agility in defending itself against invading agents—whether dust or carbon particles, microbes, or toxins—and its ability to recognize and reject tissues, cells, or chemical compounds that seem to be stamped "not self" are awesome. However, the body cannot discriminate in a given instance between harmful foreign objects and those that may be helpful (e.g., organ transplants, donor blood, medication). The body's defense systems sometimes mistake the body's own tissues as foreign and attack them; sometimes they are sluggish ("low resistance") in routing enemies; sometimes they are confused or overwhelmed by intrusions; and they sometimes mount an overkill attack that can be more harmful than the unwelcome guests.

The mechanical and chemical barriers to penetration by disease-causing agents, or pathogens, is one level of the body's defense mechanism. The surface of the skin in particular, as well as the surfaces of the mucous membranes, are formidable physical barriers to penetration by pathogens. Other mechanical defenses include the washing-out action of tears, saliva, and urine; entrapment by hairs and mucus; and expulsion by coughing and sneezing. Chemical barriers against pathogens include the acidity of the skin, stomach, and urine; and enzymes in various bodily secretions that break down the pathogen.

These mechanisms are front-line defenders; but they may fail, and pathogens may then penetrate to deeper tissues of the body or into the blood. The immune-response system then comes into battle; it is the body's internal army against both intruders and defective self-parts (e.g., worn-out cells, malignant cells, cells harboring viruses).

Central to the immune responses are the white blood cells; their actions and interactions were briefly described in chapter 1. An effective immune response by the white blood cells requires: (1) surveillance by lymphocytes and mobility of all white cells; (2) differentiation of all white cell types into functionally mature cells with normal internal dynamics, normal cell surface "announcements" and receptors (both types of structures usually being proteins or proteins complexed with carbohydrates), and normal responses to stimulatory or inhibitory signals; (3) discriminatory recognition of foreign or aberrant cells or smaller molecular structures; (4) the ability to follow effective sequencing steps or interactions that lead to elimination or inactivation of abnormal cells or structures; (5) the ability to proliferate, through cell division and feedback signals to marrow stem cells, to produce more of their kind as needed to sustain an attack, and, equally important, to accept negative feedback to stop multiplying; and (6) the capacity to age, signal their own decline, and summon macrophages to engulf them, or simply disintegrate into component parts.

These processes are carried out in cautious but rapid biological steps, with safeguards all along the route. Many activities are carried out simultaneously; it is estimated that the average cell orchestrates 20,000 reactions at any given moment. Most leukemic cells have none of the above capabilities, except the ability to proliferate.

Substances that regulate white blood cell activities—by signaling yes or no, more or less, faster or slower—include those common to many other cells, such as hormones (to which the lymphocytes are particularly sensitive, especially the prostaglandins and corticosteroids); vitamins (white cells seem to be particularly influenced by folic acid and vitamin A); interferons (which will be discussed in chapter 5); enzymes; and inflammation mediators that make blood and lymph vessel walls more porous (e.g., catecholamines, histamine, serotonin). Also important in cellular regulation are the import and transport, as well as storage, of supplies of important small molecules. Critical chemicals in this category include nucleotides, calcium, and fatty acids, whose balances at particular moments may tip the cell into a new phase, such as growth or quiescence, or stimulate or inhibit specific activities.

Other regulatory agents important to white blood cells are those largely or entirely specific to the immune system, and most of them are large molecules, usually proteins or protein-carbohydrate complexes, known as glycoproteins. These products include antibodies, produced by mature B cells (usually called plasma cells); an eleven-protein group, known as complement, whose cascade of actions, triggered by "engaged" (i.e., already coupled to antigens) antibodies, includes physical attack on the targeted intruder and summoning granulocytes for mop-up operations; a class of proteins produced by T cells and known as lymphokines, which can kill foreign cells directly, attract phagocytes (i.e., the scavenging monocytes, granulocytes, and macrophages), and stimulate other lymphocytes; and the products of macrophages, which include prostaglandins and interferon, believed to inhibit malignant and virus-infected cells.

Target-specific immune responses by the body often take place in the blood or lymph system (with its entrapment centers), but, as noted earlier, white blood cells can pursue prey into the tissues, aided by the inflammation mediators. These responses are mobilized by the presence of substances, cells, or organisms that are perceived as different and dangerous through their display of peculiar markings or signals. Their structure, or products, if they make any, stamps them as antagonistic to the host, as far as the white blood cells are concerned. Material composed of strings of amino acids or nucleic acids predominates among the possible offenders sniffed out by the white blood cells.

Because genetic information varies—not only from species to species but among individuals, certain ordered proteins will often differ, although sometimes only slightly and in ways that do not excite an immune response. But strange proteins in the context of a cell—on its surface or secreted by it—are often strong stimuli for an immune response.

These strange proteins (carbohydrates, fats, and the myriad small organic and inorganic molecules are not very interesting to the immune system) are termed antigens, and they can be considered identity markers comparable to fingerprints; in the case of a cell, the term antigen usually refers to proteins or glycoproteins displayed on the cell's outer membrane. Certain free antigens are nonetheless attractive to B cells, and call up the synthesis of antibodies.

Strictly speaking, the term antigen includes, as part of its definition, the requirement that the identity markers stimulate a response by a host's immune system, most commonly binding by T cells (i.e., the T cell locks onto a portion of the antigen), and the production by plasma cells (mature B cells) of antibodies that chemically stick to the antigen. In this sense the term antigen can be compared to the term defendant in legal usage: only when an action is brought against someone or something does the person or organization become a defendant. In our case, the host is the plaintiff and the antigen is the defendant—with a difference: this defendant is prejudged guilty.

Because a B cell differentiates into an antibody-producing cell only in the presence of antigen, it was deduced, and accepted by scientists until fairly recently, that a particular antigen's structure dictated the formula for the responding B cell's reactive antibodies. This is the lock-and-key theory, with the antigen serving as the lock and stimulating the production of a key. This theory is now controversial; and it is believed by many scientists that the fit of the key is by trial and selection. That is, gene sequences in B cells allow for any one of an estimated 1 million final "key" variations to be chosen, and only that B cell that chooses the right combination will react with the antigen, and proliferate into a clone of antibody-producing cells. In this modified lock-and-key theory, there is no customized fit; if one of the keys being made fits, it is used.

There is even less certainty about the way that T cells are activated by a particular antigen; but it is known that those T cells that do respond to a chemically attractive antigen carry a receptor that specifically allows them to combine or interact with it. It is known also that the antigen structures that attract T cells are larger and more complex than those that attract antibodies (which often respond to only a small portion of an antigen molecule—perhaps only five or six linked amino acids).

The elimination of an aberrant or foreign structure, whether it is a scrap of foreign RNA or a whole malignant cell, often begins by calling up what scientists term the primary response, which centers on antibodies. The primary response takes place in minutes to several hours, and requires the participation of the blood proteins known as complement, and the follow-through response of granulocytes that gobble up offending structures that are flagged by clinging antibodies and complement proteins. Slower to arise but often more efficient is what scientists term the secondary response, orchestrated by T cells. The secondary response takes place sometimes in concert with the antibody response, but occurs particularly if the antagonist is a whole cell. This response involves collusion between the T cells and macrophages, which provide the follow-through by gobbling up any cell flagged by a clinging T cell.

Vaccination reactions and allergies are familiar manifestations of the immune response, and demonstrate the double-edged sword that the immune response can carry. Sometimes the reaction is helpful, providing resistance to a disease (through the "memory" of descendants of once-activated B and T cells), and the effect is desired as "immunity"; at other times the same response may produce injury to a person's own tissues, through overreaction to antigens such as dust or pollen, a condition referred to as "hypersensitivity." Even more serious are the immunologic perversions known as autoimmune diseases, in which a person's immune system attacks its own tissues, misreading cellular identity markers as foreign; this situation is now known to be involved in diseases such as myasthenia gravis, lupus erythematosus, rheumatoid arthritis, and probably multiple sclerosis and a few other neurological diseases.

An immune response involves cellular interactions, synergistic activities, the release of stimulatory products, potent chemical aids (e.g., inflammatory mediators, complement, lymphokines), the guidance of lymphocytes, and the phagocytic activity of granulocytes and macrophages. The spectrum of immune-response activity is perhaps best presented, not in all its possibilities, but in a typical scheme of an effective immune response (see Figure 11):*

1. A blood protein attracts the attention of a B cell, which perceives a particular linkage of the protein's amino acids as peculiar or "not-self." The B cell is activated, usually with the aid of a "permission" protein released by a nearby T cell, a signal that it too perceives the amino acids as suspect.

2. The B cell differentiates into a plasma cell, genetically "permitted" to encode antibodies, and expresses a particular gene that "completes" its antibody so that it fits the amino acids. The com-

---

* In Figure 11 (page 62), antibodies are described as: immunoglobulins, which is the "generic" term for a family of defensive proteins, whether released into the blood (antibody) or not.

pleted antibody binds to the foreign amino acids, which are now by definition an antigen.

Antibodies are synthesized in steps; there is a "constant" portion that is the same for all antibodies of a particular class (there are five in all, called M,G,A,D,E), and a "variable" portion dictated by the gene selected to complete any particular antibody. It is the variable gene that makes the antibody specific.

3. The antibody-antigen bondage attracts the blood proteins known as complement, and they coat the antigen with parts of their own chemical structure.

4. The antibody-antigen-complement combination activates a phagocyte, usually a granulocyte or a macrophage, which will engulf the entire offensive structure, whether a whole cell or a molecule.

5. If the phagocyte is a macrophage, it digests most of the offending structure or organism; but it often spits out antigen products, which, in association with the macrophage, attract the interest of T cells.

6. The T cells are stimulated to proliferate. This causes B cells to pay attention to these ejected bits of antigen, to see if they can produce an antibody that matches any of this refuse on or near the macrophage.

7. If the antigen structure is large enough to provoke the combative interest of a T cell, and if that T cell has a surface structure (a protein) that can mesh at some point with the antigen, the T cell itself will bind to the antigen (or rather another just like it, since our initial hypothetical antigen has been engulfed). The T cell will then seek to disrupt the enemy structure (see Figure 12), and will release lymphokines, protein molecules that attract macrophages for engulfment proceedings.

8. Stimulatory or activational products secreted by the macrophage and the T cell call in other T cells, B cells, and NK cells—particularly if the antigen is part of a cell, such as a malignant or virus-harboring

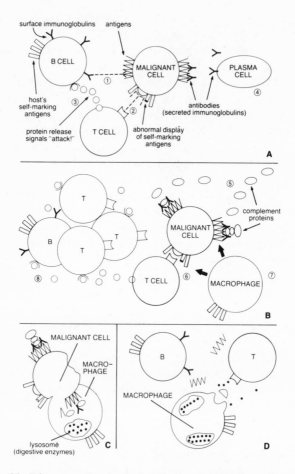

Figure 11. Diagram of a typical scheme of immune response. A B cell is attracted to an antigen on a malignant cell (A-1); a T cell is attracted to an antigen that is enhanced for recognition in the context of abnormal self-marking (histocompatability) antigens on the malignant cell (A-2). The T cell releases proteins that stimulate the B cell (A-3) to differentiate into an antibody-producing plasma cell (A-4). The catalytic and inflammation-linked blood proteins called complement are attracted by the antigen-antibody complexes and hook on (B-5). The T cell has bound itself to its target antigen (B-6). These linkages attract a macrophage (B-7). The T cell continues to release activation proteins that attract other B and T cells to the scene. The macrophage begins to devour the malignant cell, breaking it down with digestive enzymes contained in internal structures called lysosomes (C). The macrophage continues to spit out fragments of the digested cell's antigens for long periods of time (D), to warn and "teach" other B and T cells. *(Harvey Offenhartz, Inc.)*

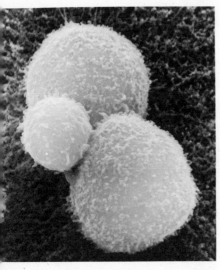

Figure 12a. A photograph taken with a scanning electron microscope, at a magnification of 9,000 times, shows one "effector" or "killer" T cell in contact with two malignant cells (the larger cells). This is a cell-mediated (T cell) immune response; and the lymphocyte is specifically stimulated by certain antigenic structures on the surface of the malignant cells that correspond to certain of the T cell's receptors *(Andrejs Liepins, Ph.D., and Ronald B. Faanes, Ph.D.)*

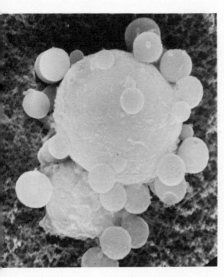

Figure 12b. A few minutes later, with continued binding by the T cell, the malignant cells begin to shed from their membranes small fluid-filled sacs, or blebs; these blebs also stick to the T cell, suggesting that they bear the lymphocyte-attracting, antigenic structures of the malignant cells. This shedding of blebs that bear antigens which correspond to the T cell's receptors may be part of the escape mechanism used by malignant cells; in effect, they are "throwing bones" to the killer T cell, in an effort to break away without attracting other T cells. *(Andrejs Liepins, Ph. D., and Ronald B. Faanes, Ph.D.)*

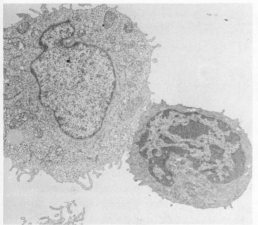

Figure 12c. A transmission electron-microscope photograph of a killer T cell in contact with a malignant cell (larger) shows a cross-section view of the surface interaction between the two cells. While there is no apparent structural disruption of the malignant cell, such as would occur under macrophage attack, the chemical message being transmitted by the T cell can kill the malignant cell within ten minutes—if contact is not broken. *(Andrejs Liepins, Ph.D., and Ronald B. Faanes, Ph. D.)*

one. If the antigen is attached to a cell, either these immune-response activities will fatally disrupt the cell's equilibrium, causing it to burst or disintegrate, or the entire cell will be engulfed by a macrophage.

9. Negative-feedback (inhibitory) signals prevent an immune response from turning into a rampage: at the same time as an immune response gets underway, concurrent "cease and desist" signals are released by activated granulocytes and macrophages; these signals inhibit activation of nearby phagocytes and travel to the marrow to inhibit overproductivity by myeloid stem cells of more granulocytes and macrophages. Certain T cells known as suppressor cells are active as well. Although this dualism may seem puzzling, the negative signals become dominant only when there are no more stimulatory signals— when there is no further exposure to antigen. In the absence of further provocation, a specific immune response usually subsides in three or four weeks, governed by the control mechanisms mentioned, and others as well.

The Genetic Factor in Immune Response

Recent advances in the field of immunology are daily shedding light on abnormalities in immune response which bear on numerous diseases, as well as on the normal process of immunologic surveillance which detects and eradicates all abnormal variants among cells, especially cells that have undergone malignant transformation. During the past ten years, genetic mapping, along with increased understanding of the complex balances and interactions of the immune-response system, have led to recognition of an immunologic element in resistance to malignancy—a factor that may be largely genetically determined.

The first medically significant genetic categorization of human beings that was made was by blood group—A, B, AB, or O. Later genetic studies, prompted by the phenomenon of host rejection of transplanted tissues, led to the recognition of another stable scheme of separate groups among humans, tissue transplantation groups. These genetically determined types get their "identity papers" (in the form of characteristic cell-surface markers) from a region on the sixth chromosome called the major histocompatibility complex (MHC). Because these cell-surface markers so readily induce an immune response if cells are given to an MHC-mismatched host, scientists often call them "MHC antigens."

Everybody has a set of MHC antigens (usually proteins, or a combination of proteins and glycoproteins) that stamps virtually all his or her cells. In addition, there is a discrete set of MHC antigens that appear, as far as is presently known, primarily on B cells and on perhaps a third of all macrophages. This subset of discrete MHC antigens appears to be critical in guiding T cell reactions in an immune response: when antigens are flagged by activated B cells or macrophages bearing the "badge" of the subset MHC markers, T cells become raging killers of the "fingered" molecules or cells.

MHC-antigen matching between donor and recipient is important in any anticipated tissue transplant; but, within the context of our concern with leukemia and leukemia treatment, the significant application is the bone marrow transplant (see chapter 3). Inheritance for the MHC chromosomal region is Mendelian; and

25 percent of siblings are therefore identical for these MHC antigens (see Glossary, "Mendel's law").

Ongoing intensive investigations suggest that genes in the MHC region are intimately linked with an individual's capacity for immune responsiveness. The genetic MHC packet which an individual receives evidently has a strong bearing on disease resistance or vulnerability, numerous specific mechanisms of immune responsiveness (e.g., "eagerness" of antibody formation and attachments by complement proteins), and, in all probability, on interactions among white blood cells—such as the vitality of macrophage-lymphocyte interactions. It has been noted in mice that different MHC codes carry predictable differences in susceptibility to virus-induced leukemia. It is known also that there are DNA segments in the MHC code for components of the complement proteins, so vital in implementing an antibody-instigated immune reaction; leukemic patients often lack, or have a low level of, certain complement components.

A connection has been established between certain MHC antigens and susceptibility to specific diseases. Over fifty MHC antigens have been characterized so far; and over eighty diseases have been linked to either an increased number of a particular MHC antigen (as compared to the number for the general population), or a decreased number. Acute lymphocytic leukemia is one of these diseases; it is linked with larger quantities of particular MHC antigens on cells, as compared to those on cells of healthy persons.

Although MHC-antigen inheritance is Mendelian, most of the eighty diseases associated with MHC-antigen peculiarity do not follow the Mendelian pattern reliably. Diseases linked to MHC-antigen peculiarity include Hodgkin's disease, myasthenia gravis, lupus erythematosus, rheumatoid arthritis, multiple sclerosis, psoriasis, ankylosing spondylitis, Reiter's syndrome, Graves's disease, chronic hepatitis, childhood asthma, juvenile-onset diabetes, and sarcoidosis.

Malignant cells usually (and perhaps always) display cell-surface markers that categorize them as peculiar or aberrant (e.g., overabundance of an MHC antigen, anachronistic structures such as "fetal" proteins, mutation-dictated proteins, viral or other frankly foreign proteins). These abnormal displays should subject them to destruction by the immune-response system. Studies indicate, for example, that the lymphocytes of almost every patient with almost any tumor are reactive against the patient's own tumor cells in laboratory dishes. In the patient's body, however, the interplay among white blood cells suffers gaps, or stimulatory signals needed to keep the work in progress are lacking.

The blame for these deficiencies cannot be put simply on the genetically "weak" or incomplete immune response in individuals in whom malignant cells proliferate unchecked. One view is that those malignant cells that survive ultimately to proliferate can successfully obstruct, inhibit, or evade a complete immune response. The qualities of malignant cells that help them avoid destruction will be discussed in the following section.

How Leukemia Cells Can Evade an Immune Response

A cell that cannot communicate intelligibly (in cellular terms) must present a great puzzlement to other cells, including the white blood cells. These obtuse cells would normally not be tolerated even if they did some things right; the maintenance of the body's integrity would require that they be eliminated. Leukemic cells have a number of qualities that either help them gain a reprieve from normal immune-response components, defraud those components, or avoid them:

1. Malignant cells are often immature in appearance and function. Even mature cells, when transformed into malignant ones experimentally, most often regress into a fairly undifferentiated state, and no longer make the products that identify them, that allow them to receive biochemical messages, or that spur their passage through the normal stages of maturity. Their perpetual infancy prevents them from stopping reproduction, and from moving through maturity into the deterioration of aging—which is flagged in normal cells by a worn-out display of surface markers that invites engulfment by macrophages.

2. Although leukemic cells usually carry malignancy-

linked antigens (fetal proteins, etc.), these antigens may be fragile or presented in an unassertive way, or may break down into simpler form: such antigens, even if they summon antibodies, may not attract the full cascade of immune-response components. The implemental complement proteins, for example, are known to require a "correct" display of cell-bound, antigen-antibody linkage. In fact, a number of investigators believe that this weak display of antigens may merely tie up the antibodies, and actually protect the leukemic cells from more avid and complete immune reactions.

3. The malignancy-associated antigens are often mobile on leukemic cells (whereas on normal cells surface proteins are firmly implanted); and leukemic cells have been shown in the laboratory to respond sometimes to the presence of antibodies by shifting their antigens, or discarding both antibodies and antigens from their surface. This "dumping" can serve as a smoke screen, protecting leukemic cells from more direct attack.

4. Dispersed malignancy-associated antigens may be so numerous that they clog the receptors of normal B and T cells. Many cells seem to be stimulated when a limited percentage (i.e., 10–30 percent) of their receptors for a given substance are occupied, but paralyzed or inhibited if these sites are saturated; and studies have shown that sustained exposure to high levels of antigen leads to immunologic unresponsiveness.

5. The weak attachments that characterize the malignancy-linked antigens (proteins or glycoproteins) characterize also many of the leukemic cell's other "working" surface proteins, such as the receptors for intercellular messages and the traffic proteins, which regulate the intake and storage of nutrients. Many of these working proteins, which normally protrude from the cell surface, extend unbroken into the cytoplasm, from which they receive signals to answer

or ignore the numerous biochemical messages. It can readily be seen that when these proteins are broken or incomplete, important messages may not get transmitted into the cell, and that no internal command to limit intake is received by the "traffic proteins."

Biological theory holds that in order for a cell's assembly of structures to go forward—such as toward the goal of differentiation—certain components, such as particular differentiation proteins must be built up continuously. If any portion of the intermediate structure breaks down (such as through DNA damage), the whole structure disintegrates and has to be built up again from the beginning. Says biologist J. M. Mitchison, renowned cell specialist of the University of Edinburgh, Scotland, "It is as though the whole house falls down when there is a temporary halt in construction."*

It can be seen how leukemic cells, with missing or falling-down bridges to communication, cannot properly listen, either to external or internal regulators.

6. Malignant cells have lowered requirements for many blood factors essential for cell growth; this could allow cell growth under conditions in which normal cells would be at rest. They can also resort to biologically primitive processes for producing energy, such as fermenting glucose. These adaptive attributes of malignant cells allow them to bypass the usual formalities required for the intake of nutrients and growth.

7. Leukemic cells produce several products (in addition to the growth-stimulating enzyme attributed to viral oncogenes and natural, "turned-on" "cancer genes") that are probably related to their energetic pseudo-youth, and which in effect signal immune

---

* J. M. Mitchison, *The Biology of the Cell Cycle* (London: Cambridge University Press, 1971), p. 211.

components to leave the cells alone and give them a chance to mature. These products can inhibit adhesion by complement proteins and inhibit membrane contact with killer lymphocytes. Leukemic granulocytes are too functionally immature to release negative-feedback signals to curb division by their own stem cells, as normal granulocytes do in order to limit proliferation in the absence of a positive signal to multiply.

EXPOSURES AND DISORDERS LINKED TO LEUKEMIA SUSCEPTIBILITY

Certain hereditary diseases and congenital chromosomal defects have been referred to earlier as carrying a higher-than-average association with the development of leukemia. Among these are Down's syndrome, Bloom's syndrome, Fanconi's syndrome, ataxia telangiectasia, aplastic anemia, and certain of the autoimmune diseases, such as lupus erythematosus.

Exposure, over a prolonged period of time, to certain chemical solvents has been associated with increased incidence of leukemia. Petroleum distillates consisting of hydrocarbons, such as benzene, are particularly indicted.

Suppression of bone marrow leading to acute myelocytic leukemia has been reported following use of the antibiotic chloramphenicol and the drug phenylbutazone, used to reduce pain and fever. Previous treatment for other malignancies with drugs known as alkylating agents, which sometimes cause chromosome breaks and also suppress bone marrow production of blood cells while in use, is associated with increased incidence of subsequent leukemia.

Exposure to high levels of ionizing radiation (charged particles, such as in X-rays) or high cumulative exposure leads to increased incidence of acute myelocytic leukemia. Radiologists sustained nearly ten times the death rate from leukemia as compared to other physicians before the widespread use of protective measures. Survivors of atomic bombings also show an increased rate of leukemia and other malignancies.

However, exposure to low levels of radiation, such as those in diagnostic X-rays, even over periods as long as twenty years, does not significantly increase the risk of leukemia, according to an extensive study recently reported by the Mayo Clinic in Rochester, Minnesota.* In this research study, 300 rads (the unit of measurement for absorbed radiation) of radiation, absorbed cumulatively over twenty years, was considered the cut-off between tolerable and excessive radiation. In a typical chest X-ray, a patient's bone marrow absorbs 1.6 millirads—a millirad being a thousandth of a rad.

As noted at various points in these chapters, any carcinogens that can bind to DNA, and any other substances that can damage DNA or deform it, are capable of serving as priming agents or transforming agents for the emergence of a malignant cell. Leukemic cells are not substantively different from other malignant cells; they are generated by DNA-mutation agents or genetic disturbances that happen to affect blood cells.

"CLUSTERING" OF LEUKEMIA CASES

A significantly increased incidence of leukemia cases within a circumscribed geographical area, occurring within a limited time period, is referred to as "clustering." The high rate of leukemia in Japan following the atomic bomb explosions in 1945 certainly fits this definition.

In Japan, the triggering event was clearly radiation exposure, but medical scientists continue to be alert to reports of case clustering that might shed light on the patterning of leukemia development that is rapid and nonrandom. James F. Holland, M.D., chairman of the Department of Neoplastic Diseases at New York City's Mount Sinai Medical Center, says that "when analyses are made of all cases of human acute leukemia, clusters in space and time cannot be shown."†

* "Study Discounts Risk of Leukemia in Exposures to Diagnostic X-Rays," *The New York Times,* 15 May 1980.
 † James F. Holland, "The Acute Leukemias," Report to the Leukemia Society of America, Symposium on Progress in Leukemia, Pathophysiology and Treatment, October 1975, pp. 10–11.

This finding does not hold true, however, when analyses have been limited to children less than six years of age, reports Dr. Holland. Among this age group, "significant clustering has been found in different parts of the world." He cites three separate study series, involving a total of thirty children—twenty-seven of them under age four—in which leukemia occurred in one child and then was diagnosed in one or more others within a sixty-to-seventy-five-day period and within a distance of one mile.

The clustering of these cases, says Dr. Holland, makes the disease occurrence by chance "highly improbable"; and he notes that these case reports "are compatible with a contagious infectious origin of acute lymphocytic leukemia with maximum susceptibility in early childhood."

This is an "onslaught" type of malignancy generation, in which a gene that probably governs a growth-related product—a "leukemia gene"—is "turned on" in a white blood cell by a mutation agent, presumably a virus. It is estimated that only some 5 percent of leukemia cases are caused directly by overwhelming and transforming viral infections. A genetically "weak" immune-response system or an immature system could allow the transformed clone —the leukemic cells—to persist.

It is known, for example, that children under age four do not have normal adult levels of antibodies of the class known as immunoglobulin G (there are four others), which exhibits the most tenacious coupling with antigens among the blood antibodies. Under age four, children must rely on antibodies of the class known as immunoglobulin M, which avidly binds antigens, but often not with a strong or stimulatory attachment, such as would attract the complement proteins. Immunoglobulin G antibodies, which make up 85 percent of the blood antibodies in normal and highly immune adults, offer a much more stable binding for antigens, are attractive to complement proteins, and tend to associate with macrophages, helping to bind antigens to them. It seems more than coincidental that the peak incidence of acute lymphocytic leukemia is in patients under four years of age.

LEUKEMIC CELL PROLIFERATION AND THE LEUKEMIA VICTIM

You don't usually think about, let alone congratulate your body's attention to cellular duties. Noted biologist Dr. Lewis Thomas contemplated one day, he reports, "thinking" for his liver. He quickly decided he wanted no part of it, that he and his liver were undoubtedly better off if it continued to manage its own time schedule and activities.

In considering what can go wrong in a body that allows mutant or malignant cells to propagate, those familiar with the complexity of cellular life might be led to think that it's amazing things work so well most of the time. This can be no comfort to those of you who suffer from, or whose children suffer from, a life-threatening proliferation of leukemic or other malignant cells. But there are new beacons of understanding and hope illuminating our knowledge of cellular life and malignant cell machinations.

The new insights are dramatically aided by the instruments that now allow genes or gene products to be read piece by piece; from work with cell fusion, in which malignant cells are harnessed to do the bidding of normal ones that make useful proteins; and gene splicing, through which microorganisms are primed to produce in quantity "cancer genes" for analysis. These techniques, combined with the insights gained through viral causation of cancer in animals, will force malignant cells from the shadows. In the words of one researcher, malignant cells will soon be in focus for a well-aimed rifle shot.

The Two-Step Theory of Cancer

It is generally believed that malignancy generated in one fell swoop, as by host integration of viral genes bearing an oncogene or viral genes inserting themselves near a natural "cancer gene," is not rare among humans but is the exception. As was discussed earlier, it is accepted by most medical scientists today, based on extensive case studies involving chromosomal analysis of cancer patients, that proliferative malignancy most often arises in two stages. Scientists describe these two steps as the inductive event, a chromosomal mutation that predisposes the person to develop cancer, followed by one or more promotional events, frank mutations that lead to malignant transformation of the cell or cells. A sizable group among cancer researchers goes even further: maintaining that although the inductive event can be a genetic abnormality that is either inherited or acquired, the promotional event is always acquired, such as exposure to carcinogens.

There is no neat one-to-one translation of a genetic change into a bizarre protein or a disease state. It is now known that genes often act in concert, and that mutations may occur in regulatory genes or DNA segments that don't show up in any protein product that is observable and peculiar. (To simply record all the nucleotide prescriptions of an individual's gene-sized DNA segments will take at least twenty years, even sequencing at a rate far faster than techniques of the early 1980s allow.)

A minor distortion in DNA may or may not be overtly threatening to an individual's health, but the mutation may nonetheless set the stage for the possible development of cancer. As to inherited vulnerability to cancer, it is estimated that of the known 2,500 human traits with Mendelian inheritance patterns, nearly 9 percent have links to cancer predisposition.

Examples of the two-step theory follow:

In a case of childhood acute lymphocytic leukemia, the inductive event could be an infection which produces a clone group of virus-integrated B lymphocytes; and the promotional event could be a second infection, such as by a herpes virus, which further stimulates B cells and "deregulates" one or several cells among the clone group, turning on a growth-related "cancer gene." A genetically "weak" or immature immune-response system might be unable to cope with the rising tide of transformed, leukemic cells.

In the case of an adult with chronic myelocytic leukemia, the inductive event could be a genetically faulty immune-response system—perhaps complement proteins are lacking or peculiar; the promotional event could be a clone line of white blood cells produced through a mutation arising from "harmless" radiation or an infectious agent. Another adult may harbor a clone group of silent yet virus-transformed cells. Prolonged exposure to a chemical carcinogen may create a series of nonharmful mutant cells, until a mutation occurs in a cell already susceptible by virus coding, and frees a repressed "cancer gene." If this cell is a white blood cell, and it can evade the immune-response system, the leukemic process can begin.

The combinations are varied, and one person's inductive event may be another person's promotional event. And of course for many of us the promotional event may never occur in the "right" cells, even though we harbor mutant cells: many cells with malignant potential do not develop into a malignancy.

The Development of Leukemia

Chromosomal deletions (the excision of DNA), additions, or rearrangements (the relocation of a DNA segment elsewhere on the chromosome)—the latter happening particularly when cells are under duress to divide quickly or when they make hasty attempts at DNA repair—can lead to or cause leukemia, as either inductive or promotional events, at a particular time in a given individual. As discussed in this chapter, certain inherited diseases and congenital disorders can constitute the first strike against averting cancer. Other inherited or acquired diseases (e.g., certain of the autoimmune diseases), conducive conditions, and acquired exposures may constitute either inductive or promotional events in the genesis of leukemia.

Among the conducive conditions presently known to render an individual vulnerable to leukemia are the presence of abnormal self-marking cellular antigens (associated with acute lymphocytic leukemia); a genetically "weak" immune-response system (dictated by genes of the sixth chromosome's major histocompatability complex); lacks or deficiencies in immune-system components (many leukemic patients lack complement components, and patients with chronic lymphocytic leukemia lack active NK lymphocytes); faulty DNA repair; chemical processing that actually enhances the potency of carcinogenic by-products, allowing them to bind to DNA; relative passivity in response to viral penetration of cells; and vulnerability to mutation from low levels of radiation or carcinogens.

Leukemia is the result of unchecked or overwhelming errors in the normal DNA sequencing that governs cellular products, or in the DNA segments that control (i.e., act as on-and-off switches for) such structural genes. According to the most recent and detailed analyses of the conversion of a normal cell into a leukemic one, a single enzyme product of one normally repressed gene can cause the cell to revert to a primitive state of uncontrolled reproduction. Or occasionally, as demonstrated in certain animal leukemias, a virus which has previously stolen one of these "cancer genes" may introduce it into a host cell, giving that cell a double dose of the pivotal gene, which may quickly overwhelm the cell with commands to multiply.

As emphasized earlier, leukemia is the result of this atavistic error in a blood cell (or genetic addition to it) only if the individual's immune-response system fails to detect the leukemic cells, or fails to effectively follow through all the steps leading to eradication of the leukemic cells. One possibility not mentioned previously is a situation in which antigen competition occurs. If an evasive leukemic cell initially arouses only a tentative antibody response, or attracts a "smoke screen" of antibodies only, and an unrelated, virulent (and "attractive") antigen appears in quantity, the lymphocytes and phagocytes may well have a higher affinity for the new peril, giving the malignant clone time to become established.

The Leukemia Victim

The individual who develops leukemia most often has sustained a double blow to a single blood cell or blood cell line; the first strike against him or her may have been a genetic dowry that includes a mutation present in all cells, or the inductive event may have been an acquired mutation, following, perhaps, an otherwise inocuous viral infection. The precipitating damage to the blood cell (or cells: sometimes separate clones are involved, derived from different blood cells) can arise from various environmental exposures, particularly those that cause chromosomal breaks, or from certain drugs, or idiosyncratic processing of chemicals, toxins, or sometimes hormones.

Following its private impulses, the leukemic cell will divide to form a clonal cluster—cells exactly like the original. Either because there is a lack or deficiency in the affected individual's immune-response system, or because one or several cells among the leukemic clone have modified their "appearance" in a way that disguises them, or sometimes because competition has arrived that is more inviting to the immune-response system, a leukemic clone becomes established. It is estimated that human leukemic cells have a doubling time of about four days; and calculations indicate that it would require about 160 to 170 days for one leukemic cell, doubling every four days, to reach one trillion—the number estimated to be lethal in humans.

By the time most cases of leukemia are diagnosed, the leukemic clone has usually become the predominant white blood cell. As mentioned in chapter 1, in such cases red blood cells and platelets are usually low in number, as are normal numbers or varieties of other white blood cells. The leukemic process seems not only to crowd out normal blood cells but to suppress normal stem cells. Researchers at New York City's Memorial Sloan-Kettering Cancer Center have recently found a common product made by leukemic cells from patients with various types of leukemia, including myelocytic and lymphocytic leukemias (with particularly high levels in patients with acute disease); this product was observed, in laboratory dishes, to inhibit directly the proliferation of normal stem cells but not the stem cells of leukemic patients. The researchers are in the process of characterizing this product.

Although medical scientists may not yet fully understand the sequence of events, and the relative amounts of influence of the various factors that can lead to the occurrence of leukemia, we have tried to explain, in this chapter, how it can happen. Individual genetic endowments and lifetime genetic revisions, environmental exposures, and ineffective or faulty immune responsiveness are all firmly implicated, and probably play interrelated roles in the genesis of leukemia.

For our readers who are leukemia patients, one battle has been lost. Your second line of defense, medical treatment for leukemia, requires much fortitude from you; and a detailed description of current treatments is provided in the next chapter. Chapter 5, "Research Directions," describes what techniques are likely to be used in the fight against leukemia in the near future, as well as the new treatments undergoing evaluation now; and we hope the survey of these advances brings encouragement to you.

CHAPTER THREE

TREATMENT

In this chapter, we will attempt to sort out what must seem to our readers who are leukemia patients, or to those who are parents of a leukemic child, a bewildering array of medical attentions. We'll describe the types of treatment, the reasoning behind their use, and what you can expect from those treatments selected for you—in terms of limitations and side effects, as well as benefits.

The treatment of leukemia is aimed at eradication or marked reduction of the leukemic cell population, maintenance of the arrested state (which can graduate into a cure), and the restitution of normal blood cell formation in the bone marrow. Current treatment centers on the use of drugs. This is known as chemotherapy (chemo = chemical, in Greek). These anti-cancer drugs come from about seven different drug categories; patients are usually given several different types of drugs in combination, in order to attack the leukemic cells in a number of different ways at the same time.

The objective in treating the acute leukemias is to kill all the leukemic cells as early as possible—before any of them modify their habits to become drug resistant. The objective in the chronic leukemias, where cell multiplication is more sluggish and erratic, and leukemic cells are therefore less reliably "open" to taking in chemicals, is to produce a daily reduction of the leukemic cell population, unless total eradication is possible.

Along with wiping out leukemic cells, current therapy emphasizes the importance of supporting the patient through the consequences of the disease process and its complicating disorders—which essentially involves boosting a deficient immune-response system and supplementing or replacing other needed blood components. This supportive care is necessary also, in many cases, to offset the effects of chemotherapy, which initially must perpetuate the deprived blood-cell condition in order to kill leukemic cells.

Surgery is not a primary treatment in leukemia, because the disease is not localized but systemic. In some cases, where leukemic cells are found to be clumped in large numbers in accessible and nonvital organs (e.g., lymph nodes, spleen), surgery may be performed to relieve the patient of this bulk accumulation and give other treatments a better chance of success.

The strategy of treatment involves: (1) inducing a remission, i.e., apparent absence of leukemic cells or the presence of only a small percentage, usually accepted as no more than 5 percent; (2) maintaining the remission; (3) reinforcing the remission; (4) treating possible or apparent central nervous system infiltration by leukemic cells (usually pertaining to the acute leukemias); and, on an investigational basis, (5) administering immunotherapy— treatment to modify or stimulate the patient's immune responses.

Besides chemotherapy, primary treatments (i.e., those intended to be the principal means of destroying or replacing leukemic cells) may include bone marrow transplants, and aggressive types of immunotherapy (e.g., interferon and monoclonal antibodies— both given to boost patients' immune reactivity against malignant cells); the latter is used experimentally today mainly for patients unlikely to have—or proven not to have—a successful response to chemotherapy. Chemotherapy and this type of immunotherapy are intended to destroy leukemic cells; bone marrow transplants are intended to replace them with normal cells, after a brief "blitzkrieg" of chemotherapy and radiation, or radiotherapy, to destroy all of the blood cells—all of which must be considered as suspect.

Secondary or adjunct treatments may include radiotherapy against suspected or apparent leukemic cell invasion of the central nervous system, or against bulk accumulations of leukemic cells in specific tissues or organs; various types of immunotherapy; surgery; and supportive therapy.

All these categories of primary and secondary treatment—including when and why they are used—will be described later in this chapter, or more completely in chapter 5 if they are being used on an introductory or experimental basis.

Patient need, combined with the probability of success and an evaluation of individual stamina and resilience, determines the range of primary and secondary treatments used. It is probable, for example, that a given patient with acute lymphocytic leukemia will need only chemotherapy, possibly preventive radiotherapy against involvement of the central nervous system, and supportive therapy. A patient with chronic myelocytic leukemia that is entering an acute phase, on the other hand, could conceivably be given, at one time or another, all forms of primary and secondary treatments.

Why these differences? It would seem that a brief and aggressive treatment would be the best in terms of eradicating the disease and allowing normal marrow stem cells to replenish the marrow and blood. This is essentially the method used with the acute leukemias, where total destruction of leukemic cells with powerful doses of drugs is attempted.

This method has been largely successful with acute lymphocytic leukemia. It has been much less successful with acute myelocytic leukemia, for reasons which are uncertain, but which may stem from the fact that acute lymphocytic leukemia is usually monoclonal, meaning that all the leukemic cells derive from one abnormal lymphoid stem cell; while the leukemic cells in acute myelocytic leukemia are often of different myeloid types (e.g., granulocytes, red blood cells) and have been shown to be sometimes of different progenitor-cell origin. The treatment of the chronic leukemias is unsatisfactory for yet other reasons.

One of the main problems in successfully treating the chronic leukemias is that, ironically, because the leukemic cells are multiplying less feverishly, a number of them are likely to be "resting," or inactive, and are therefore indifferent to chemical morsels— which anti-leukemic drugs are designed to resemble—that tempt only reproductive cells. At the time treatment is begun, the bone marrow is usually filled predominantly with leukemic cells, and any normal stem cells that remain are likely to be in an inactive state. This is the essential difference that forms the rationale for chemotherapy of leukemia—the difference between leukemic (active) and normal (inactive, or, more accurately, not in reproductive cycle) blood cells and blood stem cells. A cycle-active ("in cycle") cell is much more likely to take in "attractive" energy or building chemicals—even those laced with poisons or paralyzers. The most effective types of chemotherapy exploit this difference: they kill or paralyze cycle-active cells because they are active, not specifically because they are leukemic.

In cases of chronic leukemia, the malignant cells must primarily be attacked with cell poisons, which have little basis for discrimination. For this reason, the chronic leukemias are difficult to arrest; dosages strong enough and given long enough to kill all the leukemic cells would kill also all the blood and stem cells, and eventually kill the patient. An additional obstacle is often that patients with chronic leukemia are usually older and their normal stem cells less resilient, in terms of replenishing the marrow and blood with normal cells; and during prolonged treatment, drug-resistant clones of leukemic cells are likely to emerge.

The obvious solution is treatment that is leukemia-cell specific; and this is the goal of leukemia researchers. The closest we have come to this type of "magic bullet" is the work being done with monoclonal antibodies, which will be explored in chapter 5.

The cloud of doubt regarding the success of treatment ("Did they get it all?" "Is it coming back?") that casts a shadow over patients with most kinds of cancer is readily dispelled for leukemic patients. Patients with solid tumors, which can grow slowly over a period of years, must often undergo biopsy or diagnostic surgery to check on suspicious physical signs or symptoms, or to check on masses that appear on X-ray, ultrasound, or scanner studies. This is no simple matter where deeper tissues or vital organs may be involved. Leukemia treatments, in contrast, can be regularly monitored for effectiveness simply by taking blood samples, and, periodically, bone marrow samples. Other early-indicator tests are under development that will refine treatment-patient tailoring, to be described later in this chapter.

The strategy of using different types of anti-cancer drugs in combination; the use of individual components (e.g., red cells, granulocytes, or platelets as needed) instead of whole blood for transfusions; and the provision of zealous supportive care via antibiotics for patients highly vulnerable to infections or via platelet transfusions for those susceptible to hemorrhaging are among the current approaches to treating all malignant disease that were first introduced in the treatment of leukemia patients. Leukemia research has been at the cutting edge of all cancer therapy; and each advance in treating leukemia has brought benefits to all cancer patients.

TREATMENT PROTOCOLS

Should a bone marrow transplant be given prophylactically to a patient in remission from acute myelocytic leukemia, even though the donor match is borderline and there are no indications of a relapse? Should a young patient with chronic myelocytic leukemia who has maintained, with treatment, a satisfactory ratio of mature myeloid cells to immature, and probably leukemic, myeloid cells, be given aggressive chemotherapy because his or her leukemic cells in the laboratory show an increasing resistance to current drugs? Is infusion of anti-cancer drugs into the central nervous system, as a prophylaxis against leukemic-cell escapees, just as effective and less damaging to mental functions than irradiation?

It is obvious that a much sounder basis for answering the above questions, and the many more that present themselves as alternatives in treating a case of leukemia, exists when a record of previous experience with the same situation, wide-ranging and up-to-date, can be readily consulted. The procedures and treatments—drug dosages and frequency of administration, length of initial, or induction treatment, and many other aspects of a particular patient's therapy—are standardized at most of the leading cancer treatment centers. These schedules are called protocols; and they take into account current research findings that are evaluated continuously, in a coordinated effort by medical scientists from a number of countries.

These established treatment plans are reassessed every few months in terms of results, improvements that develop in trial groups of patients, and possible use of new drugs or approaches. One such new approach involves breeding antibodies tailor-made for an individual's malignant cells (see chapter 5). This means that every patient in these treatment centers (see "Optimal Treatment Centers," chapter 4) gets the most effective treatment available today; and that his or her protocol does not depend on the expertise or opinion of any individual physician. The protocol can be followed even if you as a patient or parent of a leukemic child choose to go to another institution, or are seen by different physicians at different times when visiting a clinic as an outpatient, or have follow-up treatments back at a local hospital or from your family physician.

Investigational protocols are designed to test whether or not inclusion of, or substitution with, promising new medications, alternate methods of drug delivery, or new combinations of drugs, can add to the average duration of remissions for a particular type of leukemia; whether or not the current standard chemotherapy regimen for acute myelocytic leukemia, for example, sustains average patient-survival periods that are comparable to those achieved by chemotherapy plus immunotherapy; and whether or not bone marrow transplants during first remission yield more long-term survivors than transplants held off until signs of an imminent relapse. In short, investigational protocols explore each promising new drug or treatment approach by comparing it with the current standard, by using separate groups of patients—comparable in all medically important ways—for each regimen.

Sometimes the investigational protocols have no norm with which to compare, but seek an answer by first-time trial (there are strict regulations for this category of investigation, which is covered in chapter 5). For example, when a new drug has been proven effective, but it is not yet known whether oral or intravenous administration is most beneficial and/or least toxic, patients will be randomly assigned to one drug-delivery route or the other. Results are compared, and, if one method is better than the other, that method is incorporated into the next update on protocols using that drug. Protocols may also include new "customizing" refinements, which attempt to fit all components of a treatment plan to the particular patient.

CHEMOTHERAPY

Anti-leukemia drugs are effective because they are designed to closely resemble chemicals that coincide with the "manufacturing" needs of cells that are preparing for or are in the process of division—as many leukemic cells are; because they resemble chemical messengers that the cell is programmed to accept (e.g., hormones); or because they unceremoniously poison any cells that are vulnerable to penetration because they are in reproductive cycle—as leukemic cells are more likely to be than most normal blood cells. Drug assault against leukemia also has the bonus of proximity: the drugs operate via the bloodstream.

Dosages of anti-leukemia drugs are carefully formulated according to: maximum allowances for killing leukemic cells without damaging too many healthy ones; the tolerance and sensitivity to drugs of the particular patient; other health-history attributes of the particular patient; and, often, body size (e.g., 5 milligrams of drug per kilogram of body weight; 45 milligrams of drug per square meter of body surface).

Anti-leukemia drugs may be given in a variety of ways: as pills; or injected intravenously, intra-arterially, intramuscularly, or subcutaneously (just under the skin), or directly to a particular site—such as into the spinal fluid, which perfuses the central nervous system. The method of delivery depends upon the impact desired (e.g., concentrated and severe or diffuse and persistent), the action and clearing time of the drug, its life and potency, and considerations of nontarget tissue effects.

The patient is usually hospitalized during induction therapy for the period required to achieve complete or partial remission—usually from one to eight weeks. Maintenance chemotherapy, which is a follow-up to induction therapy, is a schedule of precautionary drug use to catch lingering or revitalized leukemic cells; in the case of a partial remission it is used to maintain the leukemic-cell-death/leukemic-cell-reproduction balance. Maintenance therapy is usually given on an outpatient basis; the dosages are less aggressive and the drugs may differ from those used in induction therapy. Reinforcement therapy with induction drugs, for a week or two every one to three months, may be continued throughout the maintenance period, which frequently lasts three to five years, for patients who have achieved complete remission, and continues indefinitely for patients with chronic leukemias or those in partial remission.

Treatment programs vary in drug usage as well as in the total protocol: some patients take longer than others to achieve remission; individual responses and reactions to drugs may dictate drug or dosage changes; patients may relapse and require another course of induction therapy; and different types of leukemias respond differently (e.g., the chronic leukemias usually require cell poisons while the acute leukemias can be enticed by fraudulent nutrients or chemical messengers). And of course, leukemia treatment is not a static situation: protocols may change as the patient's condition changes for better or for worse; a chronic leukemia may change to acute disease; and physicians may suggest and patients may choose those experimental therapies that may improve the patient's chances for remission or longer survival, or improve the patient's quality of life.

Anti-leukemia drugs were introduced in 1947 by Dr. Sidney Farber and his colleagues at the Children's Medical Center in Boston. The initial drug was a fraudulent nutrient, a drug called aminopterin, similar to the vitamin folic acid, which is crucial to the growth of white blood cells. By thus competing with a needed nutrient, the drug interfered with, rather than nourished, leukemic cells. It was the forerunner of the drug methotrexate, an effective cell-blocking agent still in use against the acute leukemias after thirty years. Dr. Farber's pioneering therapy induced temporary remissions in ten of sixteen children with acute leukemia—the first remissions of leukemia produced by any form of treatment.

Leukemic cells are mutants exhibiting an uncontrolled pattern of reproduction; and whatever the source of the permissive signal, its obedience must be orchestrated by "turned-on" segments of DNA. Many anti-leukemia drugs throw a wrench into the DNA machinery, one way or another, so that it grinds to a halt. For example, the cell poisons (see alkylating agents, to follow) are rich in electrons when they are in solution; the formation of DNA, as when it is trying to replicate itself, is known to produce molecules that easily share their electrons to achieve stability, and the cell poisons combine rapidly with these sharing molecules. (For the opposite reason—electron deficiency—potent carcinogens bind readily to the electron-sharing DNA, RNA, and proteins.)

Single-drug treatment of leukemia has given way to synergistic combinations of drugs that attack cells in different ways; some classes of drugs (e.g., those that resemble hormones) are especially attractive to lymphocytes at almost any time, for example, while other drugs are effective against lymphocytic leukemia only when the leukemic cells are in a particular phase of their reproductive cycle. The strategy of chemotherapy is to present the leukemic cell with a bomb wrapped as a present.

The cell cycle of a reproducing, not fully differentiated, cell (usually a young cell, among normal ones) is divided into a number of phases. G_1 Phase (G = growth) is a period that normally lasts about eighteen hours, during which the cell feeds and incorporates, undergoes a degree of chemical differentiation, synthesizes certain enzymes, and begins to unravel the double strands of DNA in preparation for replication. The S Phase (S = synthesis) lasts about twenty hours, during which oxygen consumption peaks as the cell undertakes all the remaining processes necessary for DNA synthesis, and completes it, doubling its DNA allotment. G_2 Phase lasts about three hours, during which the cell synthesizes enzymes and RNA, and constructs proteins. The M Phase follows—the process of mitosis or cell division, which takes one to two hours; the cell first divides its chromosomes, and then pinches itself in half to form two daughter cells. Over one cycle a cell's total dry mass—all its components other than water, its largest constituent —increases continuously and doubles by the end of the cycle; the typical spherical cell will increase its diameter by about 26 percent. The cell cycle, then, is the period between the formation of the cell, by the division of its parent cell, and the time when the cell itself divides to form two daughter cells. A reproductive cell that is not in cycle, that is "resting," is said to be in G_0 Phase.

Following is a brief description of the types or categories of anti-leukemia drugs and the ways they are believed to act on leukemic cells:

Alkylating Agents. A group of fast-acting and highly reactive compounds that includes nitrogen mustard and other offshoots of chemical-warfare agents under development during World War II. Called cell poisons, these agents were found to destroy white blood cells; they are believed to lock directly onto the nucleic acids—DNA and RNA—and paralyze the cell's functioning. These drugs chiefly attack cells that are dividing (including, often, the stem cells) but are also able to combine with cells at any phase of their cycle. They are used chiefly in the treatment of the chronic leukemias.

Antimetabolites. Drugs that structurally resemble natural biochemicals, or metabolites, that the cell needs for energy and growth. Antimetabolites were patterned after the drugs aminopterin and methotrexate, which compete with folic acid in being taken in by white blood cells, offering the cells the equivalent of "empty calories" and thereby inhibiting their growth. There are now a number of antimetabolites which resemble other normal nutrients so closely that they trick the leukemic cells—usually "greedy"— into taking them in. Once inside the cell they compete with genuine nutrients and sabotage the production of essential nucleic acids, preventing cell growth. These drugs are used primarily against the acute leukemias, although some of them are used in certain protocols to reinforce the treatment of chronic myelocytic leukemia. They act on cells in the S Phase of their cycle.

Hormones. Natural and synthetic chemicals that accelerate or suppress the growth of specific cells, tissues, and target organs. In general, hormones are believed to act against cancer by altering or reversing a hormonal imbalance in the body that encouraged the malignant cells to thrive (e.g., the female hormone estrogen helps to suppress cancer of the prostate in men, and the male androgens can cause regression of breast cancer in women). The drugs used in leukemia treatment are adrenocortical compounds (cortisone-like steroids similar to those produced by the adrenal glands) that preferentially suppress the growth of lymphocytes. These drugs are used against acute and chronic lymphocytic leukemia, and appear to block cells in the G_1 Phase, although they can also kill cells in the G_0 Phase.

Antibiotics. Chemicals naturally produced by microorganisms such as fungi or bacteria, or synthetics that closely resemble such substances, that have the ability to suppress the activity of the nucleic acids; they are effective chiefly against the growth of other microorganisms. Certain antibiotics have proven effective against the acute leukemias; they appear to bind to the DNA of cycle-active cells, altering the molecular structure of the DNA and blocking RNA synthesis. They appear to act on cells in the S Phase or G_2 Phase of their cycle, preventing cell division.

Mitosis Inhibitors. Drugs that interfere with or arrest cell division. The one used in leukemia treatment (vincristine) is an alkaloid obtained from the periwinkle plant. It is particularly useful in treating acute lymphocytic leukemia; it has been tested against other forms of leukemia in investigational protocols, but appears to offer little if any benefit. Vincristine appears to act during the G_2 Phase as well as the M Phase of the cell cycle, preventing cell division.

Pseudoenzymes. Drugs that structurally resemble natural human enzymes that cells need to catalyze chemical reactions. The one used in leukemia treatment (asparaginase) offers a nonfunctional substitute for an enzyme needed by leukemic lymphocytes to synthesize asparagine, an amino acid essential to protein building. The drug is a reasonable facsimile of human asparaginase, but is made by a mutant form of *E. coli*, a strain of bacteria commonly found in the human intestine. Normal cells can synthesize their own asparagine, while leukemic lymphocytes cannot; they take in the pseudo-enzyme rather than plundering asparagine from normal cells. Again the leukemic cell gets "empty calories"; asparaginase selectively deprives leukemic lymphocytes without harming normal cells, exploiting a metabolic difference between normal and malignant cells. The drug is effective against acute lymphocytic leukemia, and appears to act on cells in the S Phase or G_2 Phase of their cycle.

Antiviral Agents. Currently a very limited drug category of chemicals that can inhibit viral entry into cells or, as in the case of several new drugs active against herpes simplex viruses, can selectively kill or deprive-unto-death cells bearing certain herpes-linked genetic material or products. The anti-viral action of several natural biochemicals under investigation for cancer therapy appears to be closely connected to immune-response mechanisms of white blood cells, and active in feedback mechanisms that suppress the growth of malignant cells. Interferon, naturally produced by the body in small quantities, is one of these substances, and will be discussed in chapter 5, "Research Directions."

Other Synthetics. The catchall term synthetic means simply a manufactured product that does not exist in nature, formed through a union of elements. In terms of drug development, synthetics are chemical creations that resemble known plant or animal extracts or microorganism products proven to have therapeutic value. They may be "built" according to biochemical theory, and do not necessarily resemble natural products.

The design of new compounds is often aimed at innovations

that enhance known drug activity, or that do away with dangerous, unpleasant, or simply unnecessary drug components. Current explorations in genetic engineering and biotechnology are yielding a new generation of anti-cancer drugs that are based on the principle of stimulation rather than suppression. The basic strategy is to isolate, and then find ways to produce in large amounts, natural defensive chemicals made in healthy individuals in small amounts (e.g., interferon and other lymphokines, antibodies), but made in cancer patients only in insufficient amounts or not at all. At the same time, other scientists in the fields of biochemistry and biophysics are using computers to design customized chemical keys that will exclusively fit, bind, and destroy or inactivate any disease-linked substance, including malignant-cell antigens, products, and aberrant DNA segments. These new-generation drugs will be explored in chapter 5.

The anti-leukemia drugs currently in widespread use—although some of them still carry an "experimental" classification—are listed on the following pages (see Table 2). Each drug is described according to type of anti-leukemia activity, physical appearance (e.g., pill, liquid), how given, and reported side effects (discussed in detail later). Many of the drugs are listed with brand names included in parentheses, as the drug may be better known that way. Not all brand names of all drugs are listed.

Problems of Chemotherapy and Attempts at Solutions

There are several important limitations on the usefulness of anti-leukemia drugs besides the most prominent ones—lack of specific selectivity and destructive thoroughness. These additional limitations are: (1) toxicity can damage normal cells and injure vital tissues and organs; (2) resting (G_0 Phase) leukemic cells can survive for months against a drug onslaught directed to cycle-active cells; (3) certain clones among the patient's leukemic cells may modify their habits or appearance to keep a low profile, evading or resisting the drugs in use; and (4) leukemic cells can hide out in the brain and spinal fluid, due to properties of blood vessels that largely prevent drugs from passing from the blood into the central nervous system (known as the blood-brain barrier).

TABLE 2. DRUGS USED TO TREAT LEUKEMIA

Drug	Drug Action	Drug Description	How Given	Side Effects: (f) frequent, (o) occasional, (r) rare
Asparaginase (Elspar)	Enzyme, blocks cell nutrition	Colorless liquid	IV	appetite and weight loss (f), tiredness (f), fever (o), nausea and vomiting (o), allergic reactions (r), bleeding (r), liver or pancreas damage (r)
Azacytidine	Antimetabolite	Colorless liquid	IV	nausea and vomiting (f), diarrhea (o), bone marrow suppression (o), liver damage (r), muscle weakness (r)
BCNU (Carmustine)	Synthetic similar to alkylating agent	Liquid in amber vial	IV	bone marrow suppression (f), nausea and vomiting (f), burning sensation when given (o), mild liver damage (o)
Busulfan (Myleran)	Alkylating agent	Small white pill	Oral	bone marrow suppression (f), nausea and vomiting (o), sore mouth (o), diarrhea (o), skin pigmentation (r), lung damage (r)
Chlorambucil (Luekeran)	Alkylating agent	Small white pill	Oral	bone marrow suppression (f)
Cyclophosphamide (Cytoxan)	Alkylating agent	Medium or large white pill, blue flecks; or colorless liquid	Oral, IV	bone marrow suppression (f), loss of appetite, nausea and vomiting (o), sore mouth (o), hair loss (o), cystitis (o), diarrhea (r), liver damage (r)

Drug	Type	Appearance	Administration	Side effects
Cytosine arabinoside, Cytarbine (Cytosar)	Antimetabolite	Colorless liquid	IV, under skin, spinal	bone marrow suppression (f), loss of appetite, nausea and vomiting (f), cramps and diarrhea (o), sore throat (o), headache (r), liver damage (r)
Daunomycin, Daunorubicin (Cerubidine)	Antibiotic	Ruby-red liquid	IV	bone marrow suppression (f), nausea and vomiting (f), sore mouth (o), hair loss (o), fever (o), burning sensation when given (o), heart damage (r), liver damage (r)
Dexamethasone (Decadron)	Hormone	Small colored pills (pink, green, yellow light blue); color varies with strength	Oral	weight gain and facial fullness (f), heartburn (o), stomach upset (o), suppresses immune response (o), mood swings (o), bone thinning (r), raised blood pressure (r), increased thirst, urination (r)
Doxorubicin hydrochloride (Adriamycin)	Antibiotic	Red liquid	IV	bone marrow suppression (f), nausea and vomiting (f), sore mouth (o), hair loss (o), fever (o), heart damage (o), liver damage (r)
Hydroxyurea (Hydrea)	Synthetic, inhibits DNA synthesis	Pink and gray capsule	Oral	bone marrow suppression (f), nausea and vomiting (o), diarrhea or constipation (o), rash (r), sore mouth (r)
Mercaptopurine (Purinethol)	Antimetabolite	Medium creamy-white pill	Oral, IV	bone marrow suppression (f), nausea and vomiting (o), sore mouth (r), diarrhea (r), fever (r), liver damage (r)

TABLE 2. DRUGS USED TO TREAT LEUKEMIA (Continued)

Drug	Drug Action	Drug Description	How Given	Side Effects: (f) frequent, (o) occasional, (r) rare
Methotrexate	Antimetabolite	Small yellow pill; or clear yellow liquid	Oral, IV, spinal, intramuscular	bone marrow suppression (f), mouth ulcers (f), nausea and vomiting (o), hair loss (o), rash (r), liver damage (r), diarrhea (r), lung damage (r), bone thinning (r)
Prednisone (variety of brand names)	Hormone	Pills of various colors and sizes	Oral	same side effects as Dexamethasone
Thioguanine	Antimetabolite	Medium tan pill	Oral	bone marrow suppression (f), loss of appetite, nausea and vomiting (o), sore mouth (o)
Vincristine (Oncovin)	Mitotic inhibitor	Colorless liquid	IV	pains in limbs, jaw, abdomen (o), muscle weakness (o), hair loss (o), tingling in hands, feet (o), nausea and vomiting (r), constipation (r), burning sensation when given (o)

Toxicity. Among the generative and cycle-active cells that are vulnerable to chemotherapy are those of the mucous membranes lining the mouth and gastrointestinal system, hair follicle cells and, most notably, the blood stem cells and formative cells produced in the bone marrow. Certain of the anti-leukemia drugs can also damage the bladder, the liver, the lungs, or the heart; but careful patient testing, monitoring, and medication adjustment can usually remedy this. Blood-component transfusions can help compensate for the drugs' injury to bone marrow, and certain drugs (e.g., lithium) are being used experimentally to stimulate productivity of normal stem cells.

"Rescue" therapy also helps counteract toxic effects, and allows patients to be given sweeping drug barrages that would otherwise be lethal. One important anti-leukemia drug, methotrexate, has a specific antidote called citrovorum, which in effect can replace the folic acid of which the methotrexate has deprived the cells. Used to counter leukemic cell populations (lymphocytes only) which have reached a stage of rapid cell division, a large dose of methotrexate can be given to catch most if not all of these cells. After twenty-four to forty-eight hours, the antidote is given to neutralize the methotrexate action; the leukemic cells are killed, and normal cells that were not cycle-active are rescued.

Another form of rescue therapy centers on using the patient's own bone marrow, obtained during remission, to be frozen and reinfused if relapse threatens, permitting large doses of drugs and radiation to be given in a "blitz" beforehand. Bone marrow transplants will be covered in greater detail later in this chapter.

Resting Leukemic Cells. As previously described, the most effective anti-leukemia drugs act on the basis of preferential entry and damage to cells that are gathering chemicals for the process of synthesizing or division—cycle-active cells. It has been observed that leukemic cells can sometimes survive by going into a resting phase (G_0 Phase) for months; and that these cells can recover and re-enter cycle before returning to cell division. Research trials are underway which seek to chemically lure patients' leukemic cells so that they are all synchronized into synthesizing phase, which will provide a greater assurance of destruction with a follow-up course of chemotherapy.

Decreased Effectiveness. Several steps are taken to decrease the risk of a patient acquiring a tolerance for his or her drugs. One method is to blitz the leukemic cells with high doses of two drugs that attack differently, following with a third drug with yet another point of attack, all given within a short time period. Another tactic is to give steady dosages, but expand the drug categories used, or change the drug combinations, and prescribe the drugs on a schedule over a year or longer. When a patient who has achieved remission is placed on maintenance therapy, the practice often is to use drugs different from those initially used for induction therapy, to prevent cumulative toxicity as well as to provide a further precaution against drug resistance.

Blood-Brain Barrier. Alternate methods of drug delivery have been developed to reach leukemia cells that may have taken refuge in the brain and central nervous system, and are thus unreachable by conventional routes of drug delivery. Such hidden cells can continue to multiply slowly and insidiously, until they cause CNS symptoms (e.g., headache, disorientation) or gradually work their way against the current and re-enter the general circulation, signaling re-emergence of the disease after an apparent remission.

One technique to overcome this danger is to inject anti-leukemia drugs directly into the spinal fluid; another is to deliver drugs directly into the brain by way of implanted plastic tubing. Irradiation of the brain and spine may be included in the treatment and will be described later in this chapter under "Radiotherapy."

Checking Chemotherapy Effectiveness

As discussed earlier, a patient's response to chemotherapy is readily monitored in a reasonably representative way through regular studies of blood samples and periodic examination of bone marrow samples. However, efforts are being made to predict reliably drug benefit before treatment; and to evaluate the status of sample leukemic cells from untreated patients and those who have not achieved complete remission—to discover what cycle phase most of the leukemic cells are in, then check another sample after a course of chemotherapy.

In the 1970s techniques were devised that allow human leukemic stem cells—and normal blood stem cells as well—to be kept alive and grown in the laboratory, producing their singular or diverse, more differentiated progeny, as well as simply multiplying themselves, for periods of up to four weeks. Medical scientists are now refining tests in which a patient's leukemic cells can be subjected—in the lab, prior to treatment—to various drugs, to see which drugs kill the cells most effectively, and how fast.

These tests are so far highly accurate—about 96 percent—in predicting *resistance* to a drug that is being considered, through lack of cell response in the lab. However, they are less accurate—about 60 percent—in predicting effectiveness of the drug in the body, based on a positive cell suppression or destruction in the lab. This at least eliminates drugs with toxic side effects being given to patients for whom they will have little or no benefit.

A new technology of cell sorting and measuring has been developed, called flow cytofluorometry. A sample of a patient's leukemic cells are bound to, or tagged with, a fluorescent antibody, and shot through a channel so that only one cell at a time passes before the lens of a laser. Over a million cells fly past a sensor in a few minutes, and are analyzed to determine if they are in cycle, or in what phase of the cycle they are. This allows a calculation as to the cycle status of all the patient's leukemic cells in the body —what proportion are in which phase, and what percentage, if any, are resting.

This procedure allows determinations as to whether or not cycle-active drugs should be used; which ones to use; and when, and what percentage of, leukemic cells are likely to be destroyed. The same procedure can be used following induction therapy to check its effectiveness, or to check any course of chemotherapy at any time, to help pinpoint the time to start the next course of treatment. This highly promising technique is still under refinement.

Another patient-evaluation system is independent of actual drug testing on patient cell samples. Using sophisticated mathematical and statistical techniques, medical scientists are developing criteria and ratings—following exhaustive analysis of all factors that could have a significant bearing—for predicting the likelihood of remission. Significance factors include growth patterns of the patient's leukemic stem cells in culture dishes—whether the stems produce diverse progeny or unvaried clones, whether they multiply bountifully or not; infection by pathogenic microorganisms and above-normal body temperature in the patient at time of diagnosis; age of patient; platelet count; and the percentage of immature cells compared to mature forms.

One set of prognostic indicators, based on the significance factors listed above for the acute leukemias, developed at Houston's M. D. Anderson Hospital and Tumor Institute, now allows 85 percent accuracy in identifying patients likely to respond favorably to some protocol of chemotherapy. Another set of factors, applied once a patient has achieved remission, has been developed by the Houston investigators to predict whether or not that patient is likely to remain free of leukemia for a long time.

Such analysis tailors chemotherapy more closely to the individual, and gives both patient and physician as realistic a view as possible with regard to the probable treatment outcome. It also indicates at the start the need for more aggressive therapy for patients profiled as having a probable poor response to standard protocols, or the possibility of experimental treatments or a bone marrow transplant. These classification systems—and others are being worked out at other institutions—are still under development and refinement. Further detail on work in this area appears in chapter 5.

Such advances, and all others related to promising research, treatment protocols, or technology, are shared with other medical centers participating in the controlled protocols of the National Cancer Institute's coordinated program. See chapter 4, under "Optimal Treatment Centers."

Side Effects of Chemotherapy

Most toxic, injurious, or debilitating effects of chemotherapy are reversible after induction therapy is over; and most problematical or uncomfortable side effects subside on the doses given for maintenance therapy. Perhaps the gravest long-term risk to former chemotherapy patients is that of drug-induced DNA mutations and other chromosomal abnormalities, including breaks, that can lead to new cancers later in life. Unfortunately, two of the drug categories most effective against the acute leukemias, the antimetabolites and the antibiotics, have this potential, as do the alkylating agents used against the chronic leukemias.

Following is a general description of the more serious side effects you as a patient may experience while on chemotherapy; you or your family should report the described symptoms to your physician, whether you are hospitalized or not:

1. Treatment with the anti-cancer, fungus-derived antibiotics (e.g., Adriamycin, Daunorubicin) is dose-limited primarily to prevent liver overload and possible heart damage or failure. The dosages of these drugs are lowered for patients with poor liver function, since the drug is metabolized there. Although testing and monitoring of organ function are strict with patients on these drugs, individual reactions vary considerably; any signs of shortness of breath associated with heart damage, or jaundice (e.g., yellowish skin, yellowish tinge to the white of the eyes, dark urine) associated with liver damage, should be reported to your physician.

2. Liver damage can occur, although infrequently, from the drugs asparaginase, azacytidine, cytosine arabinoside, cyclophosphamide, mercaptopurine, and methotrexate. Again, any signs of jaundice should be reported.

3. Many of the drugs used to treat leukemia cause suppression of normal bone marrow production of blood cells; the ability of the patient's body to mount an immune response in case of an infection is questionable. Any known *exposures* to measles, mumps, chicken pox, other herpes infections, rubella, polio, mononucleosis, or other contagious diseases should be reported; and any such infections, *if caught*, should be reported immediately. Severe reactions to infections may cause temporary suspension of chemotherapy.

4. Marked pallor of skin and gums (possible anemia) and any abnormal bleeding (platelet insufficiency or

impairment), including blood oozing from the gums or in the urine, should be reported. (However, it should be noted that the drugs Adriamycin and Daunorubicin turn the urine red.) Aspirin, which can damage platelets, should be avoided.

5. All patients receiving chemotherapy are at risk for permanent sterility, although a return to fertility and potency does occur for some patients when chemotherapy is over (see "Chemotherapy and Parenthood," in chapter 5). A patient who is or becomes pregnant while on chemotherapy should be aware of possible harm to the fetus.

6. Hair loss, although not a threat to the physical health of patients, causes emotional pain and a blow to self-image for many patients, particularly children and teenagers. Because the hair follicles are among the body cells with a rapid reproduction rate, they are damaged by a number of the anti-leukemia drugs aimed at multiplying cells. The use of a tight headband or ice packs to the skull, applied during the administration of certain of these drugs, has been helpful in lessening hair loss for some patients. You should discuss this with your physician. Drugs that can cause hair loss include vincristine, Adriamycin, Daunorubicin, methotrexate, and cyclophosphamide. Hair loss is usually temporary, and many patients regrow hair even while on maintenance chemotherapy.

7. Additional side effects that are not dangerous, but may be debilitating, problematical or uncomfortable, will be discussed in chapter 4, "Living with Leukemia."

SUPPORTIVE THERAPY

Infection, anemia, and hemorrhage may be part of the picture by the time leukemia is diagnosed, particularly among patients with acute forms of the disease, because of the depletion of normal blood cells. This deprivation of functional, self-generated white cells, red cells, and platelets must unfortunately continue during induction chemotherapy, which is aimed at ridding the bone marrow and circulatory systems of leukemic cells, but which also can kill or suppress normal stem cells and reproductive blood cells. The hope is that some normal stem cells are present in a resting state (or suppressed into G_0 state by the leukemic cells), and that subsequent to induction therapy they will provide replenishing activity—enter reproductive cycle and generate normal proportions and amounts of blood cells.

All-out supportive therapy plays a major role in keeping leukemia patients alive, allowing them to withstand the period of vulnerability before they can again rely on their own ability to generate normal blood cells. Supportive therapy is needed first to counteract the consequences of the disease itself, then to protect the patient from the effects of chemotherapy. The degree of supportive therapy—and the type—depend on the condition of the patient: although most patients need transfusions of red cells to insure adequate supplies of oxygen to bodily tissues, many patients are not threatened with hemorrhaging even though their platelet supply may be reduced as much as 80 percent. White blood cells are not needed to sustain life but to sustain combative life, so the supportive measures are directed to protecting the patient from infections (although transfusions of granulocytes are sometimes given).

An infection could ravage the patient whose normal white blood cells have been superseded by nonfunctional leukemic cells. Patients may have a persistent or low-grade infection upon admission to the hospital; and environmental or contact pathogens during hospitalization must be scrupulously guarded against.

Species-targeted antibiotic treatment can be given if the microorganism causing infection is known or discovered following cultures and other diagnostic tests; but in treating leukemia patients, antibiotic therapy providing broad and effective coverage is begun at the first sign of an infection. This can be changed to, or enhanced by, pathogen-specific treatment when culture results are in.

Isolation of a vulnerable patient in a restricted room or in a "life island" (essentially a plastic tent admitting only sterile filtered air) reduces or eliminates exposure to infections. This is usually done only if or when the patient is in an extremely defenseless state, such as after very strong drug dosages prior to "rescue" drugs or a bone marrow transplant.

Rigorous sanitary procedures for hospital staff and visitors, and decontamination procedures for equipment or materials used by or for the patient help to keep the patient free from infection. Should an infection occur, patients now can receive, in addition to anti-biotics, "packed" transfusions of pathogen-gobbling granulocytes, available through current cell-separation techniques applied to blood donations or supplies. Such techniques (employing natural settling partitions according to weight or density, or spinning in a centrifuge) allow the separation of the blood components needed by a particular patient from a given blood unit; and allow also the unused portion to be returned to the donor. This permits more frequent donations by one or several individuals, such as family members, which are usually sufficient to support the needs of the patient.

For example, a continuous-flow centrifuge technique separates out the granulocytes, and the rest of the blood is returned to the donor. It is now possible to get as many granulocytes from one "sitting" of a donor as are contained in thirty to forty units of whole blood collected by standard methods. With regard to granu-locytes, a histocompatible (i.e., one whose MHC antigens match the recipient's) sibling donor is best, but granulocytes from other donors in adequate quantity can also usually bring significant results in controlling infection.

Component transfusions of red blood cells—upon hospitaliza-tion, if the patient is anemic, and during the induction-chemo-therapy period when the bone marrow is suppressed—are often necessary to keep levels of hemoglobin above the threshold of tissue or organ dysfunction. Red blood cells need not be matched for histocompatability as long as the general blood type (i.e., types A, B, O, and subtypes) is the same.

Preventive transfusions of platelets, to guard against hemorrhage when counts are dangerously low, are given in many cases. Plate-lets are rather fragile for collecting and transfusion; and the best survival rate in the recipient, as well as the collection of the most functional platelets, occurs when the donation comes from a histo-compatible sibling. Other donors are also of value, however, and are often needed due to the quantity and frequency of platelet transfusions required during inductive chemotherapy, before re-vitalization of the marrow can occur.

One other important supportive measure relates to the release of toxic by-products by the drug-destroyed white blood cells. The massive leukemic cell destruction caused by chemotherapy releases from these cells a waste product, uric acid. This can lead to kid-ney failure and the presence of unprocessed uric acid in the blood —with toxic effects which can range from headaches and nausea to convulsions and coma. Short-term treatment with a drug which inhibits the formation of uric acid (e.g., allopurinol) prevents these dangerous consequences.

Problems of Supportive Therapy and Attempts at Solutions

There are two major limitations on the usefulness of the anti-infection and blood-component augmentation efforts of supportive therapy: (1) resistance to or reaction against donor blood prod-ucts; and (2) "opportunistic" infections, in which some pathogens rush in where others fear to tread.

Donor Blood Products. After induction chemotherapy, a period of time—sometimes brief and sometimes prolonged—is needed for resuscitation of normal marrow stem cells and the develop-ment and maturation of the various progeny cell lines. During this period, donor blood products may be needed; yet the renewed white blood cells—normal lymphocytes and macrophages par-ticularly—may quickly become antagonistic to the foreign platelets and granulocytes, or the foreign components may simply perform in only a desultory fashion in the new host. (Not much is required from red cells in terms of cellular interaction, and they make the transitions quite readily, as long as they are matched for blood type, as mentioned previously.) Platelets clumping, without giving effective help where they are needed, is particularly a problem in the acute leukemias of the myeloid types.

Present efforts to combat these problems lie principally in at-tempts, if a histocompatible sibling is an impossibility, to make the MHC-antigen match between the patient and proposed donor as close as possible. Parents and children of a patient or a close relative may be suitable donors: sometimes good matches can be found from previously typed individuals whose records are on file and who are available. If a good match is found, it is best to use that donor on a repetitive basis.

Another route being explored is to find substances, including natural human cellular products, that will stimulate normal stem cells into productivity, or encourage the formation and maturation of specific cell types. This way a patient's own blood-forming ability can be hurried along (as opposed to relying on donor blood products), a capability that would be particularly helpful to older patients, whose stem cells often do not revitalize quickly or readily. Lithium is one substance recently found to stimulate myeloid stem cells; and it is now under investigation for leukemia patients and others. Work in this area of these so-called "biological response modifiers" will be discussed in chapter 5.

"Opportunistic" Infections. Long before any particulars were known about viruses, it had been observed that individuals suffering one form of infection from a "sub-microscopic agent" rarely contracted another infection at the same time—that is, a second infection caused by a different pathogen. It was guessed that the first infection somehow protected the individual from other invaders. By the 1940s this observation was applied in the development of antibiotics. The theory, supported by treatment results, is that certain products of some microorganisms, injected into an individual, kill or starve other pathogens, by providing enzymes that break down the new invader, or by providing the invader with "empty calories"—substances similar (but nonfunctional) to ones necessary to their metabolism.

Today there are effective antibiotics against various types and species of bacteria (as well as against some varieties of other microorganisms such as fungi, yeasts, rickettsiae, and spirochetes); but the development of antivirals is still in early stages. The nature of the problem can be compared to the overview of medicine's conquest of certain diseases: new threats come to the fore because old ones have been conquered; for example, cancer and degenerative conditions are now prevalent causes of death because old infectious diseases no longer carry us off at a younger age. Each success answers an immediate problem and increases our longevity, but it thereby exposes us to later and perhaps unsolvable problems. Antibacterials and antifungals are often pivotal in saving lives, particularly in immune-suppressed patients such as those receiving chemotherapy, but they can inadvertantly lead to contests with viruses, or to the emergence of drug-resistant varieties of the original pathogens.

Serious infections can be caused by organisms which have selectively survived hospital use of antibiotics—organisms that have modified their habits or structure to specifically protect themselves against one or more antibiotics. Drug resistance has been shown to be carried by a DNA segment or gene—sometimes a mutant gene, or a gene encoding a protease, a class of enzyme involved in breaking down structures—that can be transmitted from one strain of microorganisms to another. The presence of low levels of antibiotics can cause an increase in the number of such genes in a bacterial population and also increase the chances of such genetic snippets being transferred to pathogenic strains. In hospitals—or individuals—where more ordinary infectious agents (e.g., *E. coli* bacteria, staphylococci bacteria) are fairly routinely under attack with antibiotics, more exotic and less manageable organisms may come to the fore.

Patients who are immune-suppressed because of anti-leukemia drugs—including patients on many protocols of maintenance therapy—or those with absolute granuloycte depletion, such as many patients with acute myelocytic leukemia, frequently need protection against a broad range of bacteria; but certain fungi, viruses, and even lesser known species of bacteria can move in where they would normally be killed or inhibited by a more overbearing bacteria or an immune response. In addition, as noted, antibiotic-resistant genes may be up for grabs in an environment (including the patient's body) where antibiotics are in regular use. Infections of the abdominal organs, heart, or lungs are especially threatening to leukemia patients.

Efforts to combat "opportunistic" infections in leukemia patients involve the judicious use of antibiotics—use only on apparent need, for specific species of microorganisms if possible, and discontinuation as soon as possible. Other steps can include transfusions of granulocytes, and sometimes the laboratory synthesis of antibiotics that are a modification of the natural or original antibiotics to be used if the patient is resistant to the original.

The development of both broad-spectrum and more specific drugs active against viruses will hopefully expand. Just since 1981 several new drugs have been developed that show promise in combating herpes infections. One of them involves the use of antibodies recovered from the blood of healthy people who have had chicken pox, and is being used as a vaccine against chicken pox (caused by a herpes virus called varicella-zoster) for children undergoing chemotherapy; two others are under investigation that appear highly promising in preventing new or latent herpes simplex infections from rampaging in active form. Interferon is also being used in patient trials as an anti-herpes agent, and has shown itself effective in curtailing the ravages of chicken pox in children who contracted it while on chemotherapy. These new drugs and drug trials will be discussed in chapter 5.

Herpes infections can be disastrous to immune-suppressed leukemia patients, particularly to those who are hospitalized and undergoing induction chemotherapy or who have received a drug and radiation "blitz" to receive a bone marrow transplant, but even to some on outpatient maintenance chemotherapy. In children under treatment, chicken pox contagion can cause pneumonia 25 percent of the time and result in death in about 7 percent of infected children. An estimated 200,000 patients being treated for cancer or who are organ-transplant patients either contract or experience reactivation of herpes infections each year (chiefly herpes simplex), and about 5 percent of them die. In immune-suppressed patients, herpes infections can spread to the brain, lungs, and liver. The new anti-herpes drugs might spare the lives of some 10,000 cancer and organ-transplant patients each year.

Side Effects of Supportive Therapy

The principal side effect of receiving donor blood products—outside of obvious flukes such as infections acquired through contaminated blood—is a condition in the patient-recipient called sensitization. This occurs as the patient continues to receive blood-component transfusions while his or her own blood-forming capability is beginning to return. The resurgence of native lymphocytes may include some that set up immune responses against the donor blood components. This is not dangerous if the patient is well on the way to general revitalized blood-forming ability; but it can establish "memory" lymphocytes that might make any future transfusions of questionable effectiveness, and possibly even hazardous.

Besides sensitization, the possible side effects of antibiotic use include: allergic responses ranging from rash to shock; damage to particular organs or tissues (e.g., streptomycin can cause ear and kidney damage, clindamycin can cause severe colitis); derangements in blood cells, including chromosome breaks; and less serious but debilitating or problematical effects such as weight gain, nausea, diarrhea, heartburn, and mood swings. If patients show serious allergic or toxic reactions to any given antibiotic, they are given reduced dosages under close supervision, or may be continued on the prescription under close supervision if antidotes are available and effects are reversible, or switched to a less toxic drug with similar purpose.

RADIOTHERAPY

Target bombardment with high-voltage radiation that results in cell-destruction, called radiotherapy, is of most benefit when directed to solid tumors or area accumulations of malignant cells. In treating the leukemias, this means irradiation of pockets of leukemic cells in an effort to kill them and provide symptomatic relief (e.g., stopping tissue destruction or invasion, relieving pressure) in types or stages of leukemia where chemotherapy has limited benefit, most particularly in chronic lymphocytic leukemia. Like chemotherapy, radiotherapy is preferentially destructive to malignant cells over normal ones because of cycle activity; and bone marrow cells and lymphoid tissue are particularly sensitive, among deeper tissues, to irradiation.

Radiotherapy may also be applied to sites of local relapse following chemotherapy-induced remission; for example, to the lymph nodes, spleen, testes, ovaries, or brain. Bone marrow irradiation is used prior to marrow transplants, in order to prepare the patient for healthy new marrow by first destroying all old marrow— each cell of which remains suspect. Another approach is the use of radioactive phosphorus, sometimes used in treating chronic lymphocytic leukemia. It is usually given intravenously, and deposits itself in bone marrow—an environment favored by phosphorus. It emits beta rays that have a destructive effect, for a week or longer, on the multiplying lymphocytes in the areas of its concentration.

Radiotherapy in leukemia is most often used for patients with the aggressive acute leukemias, as an adjunct treatment when leukemic cells (detectable in samples of spinal fluid) have penetrated the blood-brain barrier, or are causing symptoms of brain or central nervous system (CNS) damage. The X-ray treatment is not painful and is given in a series, each day's session lasting just a few minutes; the total dosage given ranges between 1,800 and 2,400 rads. (The high-voltage radiation given today—with width and depth precision focusing—does not cause the skin damage that lower-voltage sources of radiation used in the past did, nor is there the old risk of X-ray scatter.)

For a while, X-ray treatment of the CNS was done preventively for children with acute lymphocytic leukemia (ALL), after it was found that almost 50 percent of children presumably free of disease later relapsed with CNS disease. Today X-ray treatment may be given for frank symptoms of CNS involvement, but is less often given as a preventive measure. In recent years it has been replaced by—for patients with ALL—high-dose intravenous methotrexate with citrovorum rescue, with periodic delivery of methotrexate directly to the CNS. The emphasis on preventive CNS treatment has contributed significantly to the prolonged remissions and cures achieved by ALL patients. Patients with acute myelocytic leukemia may also receive CNS irradiation for frank symptoms of CNS involvement, or preventive drug injections into the spinal fluid—with cytosine arabinoside the drug of choice.

Checking Radiotherapy Effectiveness

Since radiotherapy is directed to specific tissues where leukemic cells have found sanctuary, such tissues may have to be examined independently of checks on blood cells in circulation or marrow specimens (unless the marrow is the target tissue, as in chronic lymphocytic leukemia). Tissue examination for living leukemic cells is done by needle aspiration (withdrawal via syringe) for bone marrow, or by extraction of specimens of spinal fluid to check for living leukemic cells in the central nervous system. Other tissues may be examined by biopsies, scanning procedures, or radiography of the lymphatic system (in which a substance called a contrast medium is injected into the lymph system, allowing plugs of white blood cells to be identified on X-rays).

Side Effects of Radiotherapy

This section on radiotherapy will not include a "Problems and Attempts at Solutions" discussion, because there are no major problems in the sense we have used in this book—that is, problems that limit the usefulness of the treatment in attaining success. The major "problem" of irradiation is its destructiveness: obviously, vital organs, such as the bone marrow, cannot be radiated with "curative" dosages. Irradiation has been shown in the laboratory to decrease the capacity of normal myeloid stem cells for self-renewal, and to limit their repopulating potential. Irradiation in leukemia has limited aims, generally: intended curative dosages may be given if a "rescue" is feasible, as when irradiation precedes a bone marrow transplant.

Radiotherapy to the sites of treatment relevant to the leukemias, and in the dosages given, usually causes little physical distress to the patient. The irradiated areas, however, may be subsequently vulnerable to infection and immediately subject to inflammation. Another fairly common side effect of irradiation is paresthesia—burning or prickling sensations near the irradiated area. Many patients will experience a feeling of tiredness and have dry mouth after treatments; and some may have nausea or even vomiting. There will be temporary hair loss during X-ray treatments to the head; and cataract is a rare consequence. Patients receiving X-rays to the testes or ovaries will be sterile.

Until recently it was thought that X-ray treatment, in the relatively low dosages given preventively to patients with acute lymphocytic leukemia, caused no significant damage to the head or brain. However, now that long-term studies are available, because young patients are surviving their disease, consequences of CNS and brain irradiation have shown up—and are the reason for the switch, in most present protocols, to site-infusion by a drug. Follow-up of patients who received brain and CNS irradiation when they were children has turned up cases of mildly abnormal EEG's (i.e., brain-wave tracings), growth retardation, some distortion of cranial and face bones, decreased intelligence (measured by before-and-after I.Q. tests), and learning and behavior disorders.

The benefits, in terms of lives extended or cures achieved, of focused, CNS preventive treatment are significant, and few would want to risk the fifty–fifty chance of relapse without it. Trials are now underway to establish the lowest effective dosages of irradiation, and whether CNS drug treatment is sufficient prophylaxis—and what side effects it may carry.

BONE MARROW TRANSPLANTS

The transfer of bone marrow from one person to another became feasible for patient treatment during the late 1960s, with the growing appreciation of the intricate series of cellular requirements—of both recipient and donor cells—for a compatible transfer. The cells of any transplanted tissue must carry the right "fingerprints"—the self-marking antigens carried by all an individual's cells—or be attacked by the recipient's immune-response system. In the case of leukemia patients, this problem might at first seem easily solved: wipe out all the recipient's marrow so no antagonistic (or leukemic) white cells can be formed. Two problems immediately follow this solution: If the new marrow doesn't "take" in its new home, the recipient has no blood-forming capability and will die; and, if the new marrow has different "fingerprints" from the rest of the body, its newly generated white cells will feverishly attack all those "foreign" cells that make up the recipient's body. Anything in between—the presence of some donated marrow, and some original marrow—will lead to a pitched battle for supremacy among lymphocytes, with the host body being the battleground.

The new marrow must be compatible with the "old" body; the

cell markers must be the same—both the general cellular "self" antigens, and those antigen-badges carried by a select group of "insider" lymphocytes and macrophages. These general and discrete markers are highly personal, and are determined by the chromosomal major histocompatibility complex (MHC), discussed earlier. Devising recognition tests for these blood-cell antigens—to see if two people might have the same or "histocompatible" cellular markers—was crucial to successful marrow transplants.

Many early organ transplant attempts (e.g., kidneys, hearts) failed because the grafted tissue was rejected by the recipient's immune-response system. The problem specific for grafting tissue that contains immune-competent cells, which bone marrow of course does, is graft-versus-host disease (GVHD), a rejection syndrome—ranging from mild to fatal—in which the donated marrow generates while blood cells that attack the recipient's tissues as foreign. (The reason that blood transfusions can work is that donor lymphocytes—the chief antagonists—are relatively few, and will be quickly destroyed; while red cells, granulocytes, and platelets are only moderately interesting to the recipient's immune system, providing they are matched for blood-group antigens [A, B, AB, O blood types], and are only needed temporarily anyway.) Many early attempts at bone marrow transplant failed because of GVHD, which will be discussed in more detail later in this chapter.

The purpose of marrow transplants in leukemia is to provide a fresh start, with healthy and MHC-antigen-matched marrow, for patients who are poor risks for stabilization or cure of their disease by chemotherapy. At first glance, marrow transplant may seem the treatment of choice for all leukemia patients—that is, simply wipe the slate clean and start over. But the procedure itself carries significant risks, and not everyone has a matched donor—limitations which will be discussed later.

The first successful transplants of bone marrow from one person to another (termed allogenic transplants: allogenic = made by another) were done in the mid-1960s. Since that time such transplants have been done in controlled and ongoing programs at about a dozen U.S. medical centers, with the program at the Fred Hutchinson Cancer Research Center in Seattle, Washington, being the longest established. Patients include those with inherited or chronic immune deficiencies, aplastic anemia, and malignancies of the blood-forming tissues, including lymphoma and leukemia.

Allogenic bone marrow transplants, done in the 1970s in the treatment of acute leukemia, were initially used primarily to treat patients in relapse with acute myelocytic leukemia. This was because acute myelocytic leukemia is difficult to control with tolerable dosages of chemotherapy or for extended periods of time; and remissions following relapse are difficult to achieve and precarious at best. As noted previously, acute lymphocytic leukemia is usually well managed by current treatment protocols; however, some patients resistant to chemotherapy or who have suffered several relapses may be candidates for marrow transplants. Overall, these allogenic transplants for patients in critical condition and with poor prognosis have had a 14 percent cure rate—patients surviving, so far, five to ten years after transplantation.

In the late 1970s a number of medical centers began trials of allogenic marrow transplants for patients stabilized in first remission or in the earliest stages of relapse. Most of these patients had acute myelocytic leukemia or a form of acute lymphocytic leukemia—T cell—known to be difficult to control with current maintenance protocols.

The reasoning was that a treatment effective for late-stage or relapsed patients should be even more effective for patients in early stages of treatment or in remission. Patients in good general condition would have a much better chance of surviving the risks of the transplant procedure; the total number of leukemic cells the new white cells might have to eradicate would be minimal or possibly nonexistent; and any lingering leukemic cells should not yet have become resistant to chemotherapy—a high-dose blitz of which would precede the transplant.

Results to date from several centers indicate an average survival rate for these good-condition transplant patients of about 45 percent, for periods now as long as two to six years. This is significant in view of the survival rate for acute myelocytic leukemia treated by chemotherapy, which averages about 20 percent for survival past five years. Another advantage is that patients whose marrow graft "takes" usually do not need maintenance chemotherapy.

110

Bone marrow transplantation is considered investigational, in that a number of aspects of the procedure are still in trials for effectiveness or comparison with chemotherapy, in various experimental protocols; and long-term results with a sizable number of patients are still awaited. Statistics and protocols from most medical centers where marrow transplants are performed are analyzed by a central bone marrow transplant registry, maintained by the National Institutes of Health. Its data are available to all centers performing or about to undertake marrow transplant programs, both in the United States and other countries, and to physicians treating patients who may be transplant candidates.

Candidates for Allogenic Marrow Transplants

The main criterion for patients to become candidates for allogenic bone marrow transplant is that each has a prospective donor who is a perfect or close match for cellular MHC antigens. The matching tests will not be described in detail (they are still being expanded and refined); essentially, lymphocytes are used since they bear both sets of antigens of concern (i.e., the general "self" antigens plus the discrete "insider-badge" antigens), and they are cultured together to see if or where they attack each other. In an acceptable donor-recipient match, there is no antagonism, as in making preparations for division, the prelude to an attack.

An actually perfect match can exist only between identical twins, whose chromosomal inheritance is the same in every respect. Siblings of a prospective recipient have a 25 percent chance of being histocompatibly perfect matches in the tests currently available for detecting any MHC-antigen differences. Studies to expand matching tests to include "minor" MHC-antigen identity or differences are being pursued.

Most patients do not have an identical twin. Among all patients having at least one sibling, about 48 percent have a "matched" sibling. This initial hurdle obviously excludes many patients as transplant candidates. The sex of donor and recipient is not a criterion for marrow transplantation; matches can be the same sex or opposite sexes. If blood types are incompatible—which can occur even between MHC-antigen matches—a complete exchange blood transfusion must be done, except if the prospective donor is type O—the universal donor.

Other qualifications that have arisen are:

1. Patients should be in good general condition; patients with organ involvement (leukemic cell invasion), infection, or in late stages of relapse are not acceptable candidates.
2. Patients must be judged capable of withstanding the "prep" treatment of concentrated, high-dose chemotherapy and total-body irradiation.
3. Age appears related to outcome; and patients over forty are usually not considered acceptable candidates.
4. Patients presensitized to foreign antigens through numerous blood transfusions are usually not considered the best candidates, although this factor has become less important with the drug blitz that suppresses the immune response before transplantation, and immunosuppressive drugs given following the transplant.

Transplant Procedure

After acceptance as a compatible match, the prospective donor is often asked to donate whole blood, granulocytes, or other separate blood components, before the transplant, so that they are on hand for the patient later. (Following the transplant the donor may also be asked to donate blood components, as determined by the patient's condition.) The donor is admitted to the hospital the day before the marrow is taken and is usually released on the same day as the operation. The donor receives general or spinal anesthesia, and the marrow is removed in the operating room. The marrow is usually extracted from multiple sites in the hip bone (entered from the back) by needle aspiration, and between fourteen and twenty-seven fluid ounces of marrow are taken. Donor marrow is usually restored in a few days to normal amounts;

a blood transfusion may be given, often of the donor's own blood, taken previously and stored.

Protocols for prepping the transplant recipient vary, but most now include: sterility procedures for about a week before the transplant, including administration of antibiotics, to render the patient germ-free; high-dose chemotherapy from one to eight days preceding the transplant; and total-body irradiation the day of the transplant, usually at a dosage level close to 1,000 rads, and often delivered by radiation sources such as linear accelerators, instruments that deliver high-energy atomic particles such as electrons or neutrons. The prep is aimed at total destruction of all marrow cells.

The donated marrow is usually infused intravenously, just like an ordinary blood transfusion; although at some centers the infusion is directed into the heart chamber, via a catheter, or thin tube. A significant proportion of the transfused marrow cells will "colonize" the recipient's marrow spaces, where, in this appropriate environment, they slowly begin to proliferate, produce progeny lines, and reconstitute the marrow with normal proportions of normal cells. Adequate marrow repopulation, following a graft "take," usually occurs in two to four weeks.

Following the transfusion, the patient receives drugs for varying lengths of time to prevent or treat GVHD; and is kept in a protective isolation room for about three weeks—longer, of course, if needed. The total length of hospitalization averages about two months.

Protocols vary for anti-leukemia and immunosuppresive drug prepping in length of time drugs are given and type of drugs given to guard against or combat GVHD; in whether or not drugs are given preventively at all; in whether or not prophylactic granulocyte transfusions from the marrow donor are given; and in whether or not anti-leukemia maintenance drugs are given following transplantation. Most post-transplant patients need transfusions of varying amounts of blood elements—platelets and granulocytes are needed most often, red cells less often. These blood components are irradiated prior to transfusion to inactivate any immune-competent lymphocytes that could contribute to GVHD.

Cell cultures are done frequently—usually weekly, during the immediate post-transplant period, so that antibiotics can be given in the event of an infection; many patients are given broad-spectrum antibiotics routinely, as a precaution. Patients are given more intensive antibiotic therapy immediately if a fever arises.

Transplant patients usually have their diet restricted to well-cooked—and frequently sterilized—foods during the recovery period in the hospital; and many go through a period when they must be nourished intravenously, due to mouth sores arising from radiotherapy as well as the strong prep doses of drugs.

Bone marrow samples are taken several times during the hospital posttransplant period, until the "take" is assured. Donor blood elements are transfused as needed during this period. Patients with acute lymphocytic leukemia—and other types of acute leukemia as well, in some protocols—usually receive prophylactic CNS drug therapy periodically for several months after transplantation, during their hospital stay and afterward. The transplant patient remains in the hospital until the marrow graft is functional and he or she is able to eat normally, and is on the way to a return to immune-responsiveness, as demonstrated through various tests.

Problems of Allogenic Marrow Transplants and Attempts at Solutions

The immediate problem of a transplant's failure to "take" has been all but eliminated due to present-day care in selection—painstaking compatibility testing between prospective donors and recipients of bone marrow transplants. Other obstacles that may impede or prevent bone marrow transplantation from successfully controlling leukemia and leading to restored health include the following major problems:

Toxic Reactions. There is the possibility that some patients can experience severe or even fatal toxic reactions to the prep protocol of irradiation and chemotherapy, due to tissue or organ intolerance because of previous chemotherapy, or for idiosyncratic reasons that couldn't be anticipated. This can happen despite the fact that criteria for patient selection today include good general condition and no known hypersensitivity to tissue damage by drugs. The most serious toxic reactions include kidney insufficiency, liver damage, respiratory failure, and heart failure. Severe hemorrhagic cystitis, a complication seen fairly often until recently and due to cyclophosphamide, a drug commonly used in the prep for transplantation, has been averted through the use of bladder irrigation —a direct and continuous rinsing. The prep drug dosages and combinations used today are calculated to assure effective marrow-cell destruction within tolerable bounds of effect on other body tissues. Of course equipment is on hand to resuscitate any patient who develops respiratory or heart failure, although this is now an infrequent occurrence.

Graft-Versus-Host Disease. Some degree of GVHD is seen in almost 70 percent of posttransplant patients. It is initiated by the attack of newly generated donor lymphocytes against certain target tissues in the host that are known to, or may, bear cells with the discrete MHC antigens. Skin cells bear the "old"—that is, host-native—discrete MHC antigens, as do B lymphocytes and a number of macrophages, which may be hiding out in the tissues that are now read as "enemy." GVHD in mildest form results in skin rashes; it also seems to encourage infections. The more severe —or fatal—GVHD reactions include sloughing of skin, damage to the gastrointestinal tract (which can result in severe diarrhea and abdominal pain, or ulcerations along the tract), liver failure, and an overall condition perhaps best described as wasting away.

The fact that GVHD can occur even in a recipient matched with a donor for general MHC antigens indicates that the discrete MHC antigens or other "minor" self-marking antigens may be different for the two; that some as yet unknown other genetic "system" may mark certain cells that differ between donor and recipient; or even that unrecognized organ-specific antigens may differ. Currently, about 12 percent of transplant recipients die of uncontrollable GVHD, often combined with viral pneumonia.

Prophylactic drug treatment is commonly given to suppress GVHD; in effect it inhibits the new lymphocytes. Methotrexate and prednisone are the drugs often used. Other immunosuppressive drugs are added if needed (e.g., cyclophosphamide, cytosine arabinoside); and a special antithymocyte globulin (thymocytes are the new and immature T lymphocytes) may be given—antibodies that have been made by other species, such as rabbits and horses, against human thymocytes to which the animals have been exposed. Immunosuppressive therapy is often routinely given for several months, and is continued indefinitely if needed.

Infections. After marrow grafting, immune competence takes a considerable time to develop—especially if immunosuppressive drugs must be given. It is as if, as one researcher described it, the immune system were put back to fetal status and had to develop anew. During this recovery, or development, infections can prove life threatening. One of the most serious and most common is viral pneumonia (usually caused by a herpes virus known as cytomegalovirus), which is a complication in about 25 percent of otherwise successful marrow transplants. Other herpes infections are also frequently encountered; various other viral, bacterial, and fungal infections may occur.

The treatment of infections has been described elsewhere in this chapter; broad-spectrum antibiotics or organism-specific antibiotics, if existent, are given. Recently, several newly developed anti-herpes drugs are being tried on transplant patients, including prophylactically prior to transplant for patients known to harbor latent herpes infections; results are promising. Drugs that stimulate the production of granulocytes or stimulate anti-viral activity (e.g., interferon) are also being tried. These new drugs will be discussed in chapter 5.

Recurrence of Leukemia. In a minority of marrow transplant patients, leukemia may recur. In some cases the leukemic cells are identified as host-native (through analysis of MHC antigens and other cell markers), and it therefore appears that all leukemic cells were not destroyed during transplant prep, or that the "leukemic process" began again. In a very few cases the leukemic cells are identified as being of donor origin, most readily shown when donor and recipient are of opposite sex and have different sexual chromosomes (i.e., the XX [female] versus XY [male] pattern of chromosomes 23—see Figure 8 on page 37, representing a male pairing). To account for this latter situation, current theories propose that: the transforming agents are still free (e.g., virus particles, mutant DNA segments released from the degenerating host leukemic cells) and have integrated themselves into a donor cell; chemotherapy and irradiation prep prior to transplant caused new mutations whose encoded proteins have malignantly transformed the new cells; the transforming vulnerability still exists within the patient, due to genetic or other susceptibilities governing cell regulation; immune-response suppression following transplant could lead to lack of reactivity against spontaneously arising malignant cells; or that graft-versus-host reactions themselves produce leukemic cells.

Patients who relapse following marrow transplants are not generally given further transplants. They are put on standard or investigational protocols involving chemotherapy and/or immunotherapy, with supportive treatment as needed.

Many improvements and refinements will have to be accomplished before marrow transplants between other than identical twins can be reasonably expected to succeed; it is estimated that only 10 percent of leukemia patients meet today's qualifications for acceptance as allogenic marrow recipients, and the procedure carries significant risks, as outlined. The new trend toward transplants when the patient is in remission, or in the earliest stage of relapse, may offer the transplant option to greater numbers of patients—a boon if the serious and general problems of GVHD and infection can be more successfully handled.

Advances in treating GVHD and in stimulating the functioning of the immune-response system are encouraging. There is the possibility of developing a register of MHC-antigen types, to allow transplant matches between unrelated persons (done in a few experimental situations); and there will be further understanding, along with recognition tests, of "minor" cell-antigen compatibilities that may significantly improve transplant matches. An innovative approach, in the earliest phase of investigation (first case report in December 1982), uses monoclonal antibodies—quantities of antigen-specific immunoglobulins churned out by genetically-manipulated bacteria—to "neuter" MHC antigens on marrow cells of a donor imperfectly matched with the prospective recipient, so that the new cells will not initiate GVHD and will have a chance to "take" in the recipient. See the section on monoclonal antibodies, chapter 5.

Checking Marrow Transplant Effectiveness

As noted earlier, adequate marrow activity, resulting in effective blood levels of the various types of blood cells, usually occurs in about three weeks after transplant, although a normal platelet count often takes over three months. The generative ability of the new marrow can be readily checked by blood samples and then marrow specimens. Of course it is important to establish that the new cells are of donor origin, and this can be done through chromosome analysis (when the donor and recipient are of opposite sexes); analysis of red cell antigens (i.e., A, B, AB, O blood type and subtypes); or the more painstaking analysis of MHC antigens; and other differential tests as well, if needed. (None of these distinguishing tests applies when donor and recipient are identical twins.)

After checking that the patient has developed adequate levels of blood cells generated by the new marrow (that is, independent of component transfusions), the next hurdle is to establish that the patient's immune response is functional. There is a battery of tests to challenge the responsiveness of the patient's white blood cells; among them are skin tests with provocative (but noninfective) substances that should elicit both primary and secondary immune responses, and laboratory tests that will stimulate lymphocyte activity if the lymphocytes are normally reactive.

Side Effects of Marrow Transplants

One of the more serious possible side effects of a marrow transplant is that the new marrow may contain cells that harbor viruses or that contain viral genetic material. Such viral "information" could be liberated when the patient is on an immunosuppressive regimen. Another possibility is that mutant cells may be among those donated, and that the marrow recipient is less stringent about controlling mutations. Consequences of the prep treatment include the possibilities of cataracts and an increased risk of later, second cancers; and all patients are subject to permanent sterility. Less serious side effects are those that temporarily follow the prep treatment, including nausea and vomiting, diarrhea, low-grade fever, swelling of the salivary glands, and mouth sores.

Autologous Marrow Transplants: Recipient as Donor

The use of the patient's own marrow, taken when he or she is in remission and reinfused if relapse occurs, eliminates the need for a compatible donor, the possibility of GVHD, and the need for immune-response suppression with drugs. These advantages are balanced by the risk the procedure introduces—the strong possibility of returning the patient's disease along with the marrow. This type of transplant is known as autologous—coming from the self; it provides a treatment option for patients who have suffered relapses, who are resistant to chemotherapy, or who cannot tolerate effective dosages of chemotherapy, and who would die without some alternate therapy.

At Houston's M. D. Anderson Hospital and Tumor Institute, where the greatest number of autologous marrow transplants have been done, candidates are limited to those who have been in complete remission at least four months following their marrow banking, prior to the relapse crisis, thus reducing the chances of leukemic cells being in the transfusion. The hazards of toxicity due to the prep regimen, and infection following the transplant, attend autologous transplants as well as allogenic marrow grafts. Candidates are usually limited to those under fifty years of age.

As in allogenic marrow transplants, autologous grafts permit physicians to first prep the patient with high (and otherwise lethal) doses of drugs and radiation, in an effort to eradicate all marrow cells. The patient's own preserved and thawed marrow cells provide the rescue; the marrow is infused as in allogenic transplants, and the cells should repopulate the marrow and reconstitute the blood.

Techniques are now being developed that will allow a more certain separation of normal from malignant marrow stem cells, which would greatly increase the chances of full recovery for autologous transplant patients. Techniques are also being worked out to permit stem-cell harvesting from the blood, where there are normally few. This method would involve rapid cycling and return of the remission patient's blood, with select removal of the stem cells for preservation—avoiding marrow donation procedures.

With the experience gained in leukemia treatment, autologous marrow collection and preservation is being used to provide a second line of defense for patients with solid malignancies, such as breast cancer, lung cancer, and cancers of the colon and testes. If relapse or metastasis occurs, the remission marrow can be used, following a "wipe-out" prep similar to that used with leukemia patients. This procedure is now being considered as an experimental front-line treatment for patients with tumors who have a poor prognosis with other conventional means of treatment.

IMMUNOTHERAPY

Immunotherapy, a branch of medical treatment in its infancy, is concerned with getting around the weak links in the immune-response system in individuals who demonstrably lack effective defenses against disease. The two major approaches are: (1) injecting the patient with substances that will generate greater productivity of white blood cells, or that will stimulate or provoke search-and-destroy action by the lymphocytes; and (2) injecting the patient with natural, synthetic, or "engineered" substances that will override immune-response lacks, compensating the patient with chemicals that protect normal cells or attack abnormal ones.

Immunotherapy is too new to be relied on as a front-line attack against cancer. It is being used today as a supplemental treatment for patients in remission, or as an experimental treatment for patients who have a poor prognosis with other available treatments. All types of present-day immunotherapy are known to be most effective when the patient is harboring relatively few or elusive abnormal or malignant cells.

One of the first attempts at immunotherapy against cancer, and one still useful in prolonging remissions for patients with acute myelocytic leukemia, was to "vaccinate" the patient with inoculations containing another person's leukemic cells—irradiated to make them sterile—and a "tame" form of the tuberculosis bacillus (vaccines called BCG and MER). This has been found to "beef up" the immune response in some patients, without threatening the remission.

A newer approach involves giving the patient certain chemicals (such as interferon and other lymphokines) that are produced in healthy persons when the immune system is activated, in the hope that these substances might communicate an "attack" message to the patient's inert or confused white blood cells, prompting the white cells to multiply and seek out an enemy. As bait, physicians can inject a sample of the patient's irradiated leukemic cells, whose surface products or antigens will hopefully be read as suspect or hostile in the chemical atmosphere of a created alert.

A recent method of "educating" white blood cells has been to take lymphocytes from patients in remission and expose them in the lab to samples of the patient's leukemic cells, which have been chemically enhanced to invite destruction—that is, they have been made potently antigenic. The lymphocytes are then injected back into the patient in the hopes that they and their clones will recognize the enemy without enhancement, should it ever be encountered in the body, and call up a complete immune response.

Yet another teaching system involves uncloaking leukemic cells with enzymes that remove certain surface acids, fully exposing proteins on the surface that are more generally antigenic, and which will hopefully act as more potent and recognizable "foreigners." The patient in remission is injected with small numbers of these cells over a period of time; the cells are sterile, and a supply is kept frozen. This technique is being used at New York City's Mount Sinai Medical Center for patients who are in remission following inductive chemotherapy for acute myelocytic leukemia. The sensitization process takes about two years, and involves monthly injections. Mount Sinai researchers report that of the 30 percent of patients who survive the two years, subsequent relapse is rare; and remissions have continued up to eight years so far.

Chemicals that will stimulate the repopulation of bone marrow cells, and in particular the production of healthy and competent white blood cells, are being intensively investigated. One of these drugs is lithium, whose ability to stimulate marrow stem cells into productivity was found by chance through records on its use in patients being treated for manic-depressive emotional disorders.

Lithium is now being evaluated in several trials with patients who have undergone chemotherapy.

An exciting line of investigation is that of producing an extensive arsenal of monoclonal antibodies; these antibodies are engineered in the lab to be singularly selective, each batch a perfect reproduction of antibodies produced by a "master" plasma cell. The master cell in turn is primed by a specific antagonist—such as an antigen unique to an individual's malignant cells—and is permanently programmed to produce antibody against that target only. The master cells must be preserved and kept functional; and work is underway to develop strains of hybrid cells, the producers of these pure antibodies, that will be stable and durable. It is theorized that by combining these antibodies (made to any antigen specifications) with a powerful cell-killing substance, a "magic bullet" could be produced that would selectively recognize and destroy a patient's malignant cells. A description of these investigational and experimental techniques, along with the results in early trials, will be discussed in chapter 5.

REMISSION AND RELAPSE

Remission for patients with leukemia is the apparent disease-free condition brought about by chemotherapy, radiotherapy, bone marrow transplants, or immunotherapy. A patient's initial course of treatment is called induction therapy—that is, it is meant to induce a remission.

Remissions are considered complete when there are no recognizable leukemic cells in the bone marrow, and when the marrow's activity and proportions look normal. (No leukemic cells are alive in circulation, as checked through blood samples subjected, in medical centers with the equipment and expertise, to scrutiny with flow cytofluorometry.) The patient in complete remission has adequate platelets, white cells, and red cells, and is clinically well—restored to good health.

If the blast cells—stem cells or very immature cells—are less than 5 percent in the marrow, it is almost impossible with available techniques to differentiate as to whether they are normal or leukemic; and patients who achieve this normal percentage are considered to be in complete remission if the percentage is sustained. Patients who have 25 percent or less of blasts in the marrow are considered to be in partial remission. Patients with large percentages of blasts have not achieved remission.

Patients in remission are placed on maintenance chemotherapy —with the exception, in some protocols, of patients who are successful marrow transplant recipients. Maintenance therapy for acute lymphocytic leukemia patients usually consists of drugs that were not part of the induction treatment; and the drugs are taken regularly, on an outpatient basis, for periods ranging in most protocols from three to five years. Patients with acute myelocytic leukemia—and other types of acute leukemia—in remission receive periodic maintenance therapy that resembles the induction treatment, or receive courses of various drug combinations in rotation, because, as noted earlier, these types of acute leukemias are difficult to control with tolerable dosages of maintenance chemotherapy. Maintenance therapy may include some form of immunotherapy, and patients may need some type of support therapy—such as prophylaxis against infection or treatment of infection.

Patients in remission from acute lymphocytic leukemia, on the less aggressive drug regimens of maintenance chemotherapy, also receive periodic reinforcement chemotherapy in some protocols. This is a precautionary drug treatment, given every month, or every several months, often consisting of the same drug combination used to induce remission successfully.

Treatment protocols vary for patients with the chronic forms of leukemia, and for patients who are unable to achieve remission. Such patients are usually prescribed drug combinations with the aim of reducing the leukemic cell multiplication enough to provide a livable balance, within tolerable limits of drug toxicity. If chronic leukemia enters an acute stage, as often happens, it is treated with induction-type chemotherapy.

Patients in remission as well as those under other leukemia management drug programs on an outpatient basis are checked frequently by blood samples, and periodically by bone marrow samples. Relapse of leukemia can be detected in the marrow weeks or months before it would become apparent in the blood.

If large numbers of blasts appear in the marrow, along with

other leukemia-linked changes in the marrow, blood, or body chemistry, or if symptoms and tests indicate organ involvement, a patient is in relapse. This means that leukemic cell clones have again multiplied: perhaps from a single resistant cell or cluster of hidden or resting leukemic cells, or perhaps from a new occurrence of mutant-into-leukemic cells.

The patient in relapse is again hospitalized and undergoes a course of drug treatment as aggressive as the induction therapy, if it can be tolerated; different combinations of drugs may be used. The patient may elect to try an experimental drug that has shown to be promising and safe in lab and animal studies, or an experimental treatment such as marrow transplant (if feasible) or aggressive immunotherapy.

Remissions achieved through protocol programs of chemotherapy following a relapse are usually not as long as the first, and subsequent relapses are progressively more difficult to control. Therefore intensive efforts are made to sustain and bolster the first remission.

CHAPTER FOUR

LIVING WITH LEUKEMIA*

Elizabeth's sick, and she's sad.
> —a five-year-old leukemia patient
> from Ohio, at home during remission,
> describes herself

The thing I'm most happy about is that I'm living. I appreciate life more than I did before.
> —a twelve-year-old leukemia patient from
> the San Francisco Bay area

I felt my values shifting and pettiness being eliminated from my life. I'll never dread another birthday. Each one will be a gift of time, and growing old will be a gift of life.
> —a thirty-six-year-old leukemia patient from
> Connecticut, in remission following
> a bone marrow transplant from her
> younger sister

Elizabeth also had ferocious outbursts of anger—one evening tearing up everything in her room—and periods of withdrawal, when she refused to speak to any adult other than her mother. Children and teenagers with leukemia can range readily from hostility and withdrawal to an attitude of life appreciation that impresses others as "a wisdom far beyond their years," as the

---

* Books, organizations, and other sources of help and information mentioned in this chapter are listed at the back of this book.

producer of a television documentary on leukemic children observed.

They can also display defiant humor, such as the ten-year-old boy, who after losing his hair during chemotherapy, sported a "Bald Is Beautiful" T-shirt; or the young Brooklyn woman who referred to New York City's Memorial Sloan-Kettering Cancer Center as "my East Side pad."

Probably all leukemia patients periodically, and particularly initially, grapple with the "unfairness" of it all, wondering why this happened to them. And with the exception of the very young children, probably all leukemia patients have looked into the abyss, contemplating their own deaths. Their families, too, must look into the abyss of death.

The profound experiencing of life as fragile and temporary, and the acquisition of a humbling perspective on one's place in the sun, creates for many patients and their families a new spirit and insight, breeding gratitude for the small favors of life. For others it breeds a sense of diminution that results in defiance or despair.

Acceptance of one's new situation does not come easily, nor does adjustment to it. It is costly. Equilibrium must be continuously sought, won, and re-won; it is easily overturned, according to those who have lived with leukemia.

One of the first significant choices you, as a diagnosed leukemia patient, or as the parent of a leukemic child, must make is where treatment will take place. (Most patients are initially diagnosed by a family physician, internist, or pediatrician.)

The selection of the hospital or medical center where treatment will be undertaken is of vital importance; and only the best treatment is good enough to assure even odds against leukemia. The diagnosing physician may have excellent sources of referral for leukemia treatment, particularly if he or she is associated with a major medical center; or may offer a little guidance. Protocols may be standardized, but the leading cancer centers are best able to evaluate the patient, establish the most appropriate protocol, or make decisions on the use of marrow transplants or experimental treatment.

OPTIMAL TREATMENT CENTERS

The most encouraging results in remissions and lengthening survival periods for leukemia patients come from major medical centers where cancer research is intensive and staff expertise in cancer treatment is extensive. Many of these centers participate in the coordinated research and treatment program of the National Cancer Institute (NCI), which demands of member institutions highly trained staffs, cooperation under rigorously controlled treatment protocols, full support services (e.g., nursing, laboratories), and up-to-date facilities and technology.

These centers have access to the promising new drugs which are being tested under investigational procedures approved by the Food and Drug Administration (FDA). Each of these member institutions also has staff representatives who regularly communicate with, and receive patient-trial results—including treatment changes that appear beneficial—from, the NCI and the other member institutions.

There are about eighty major medical centers that are NCI member institutions. They are regionally divided into three groups: one representing institutions serving the Midwest and West; one serving the East (and including representatives from several European countries); and another serving the Southwest. These groups hold regular meetings of their member-institution representatives, at which treatment protocols are created, evaluated, modified, or discontinued.

A listing of, and information about, institutions that are participants in the NCI's coordinated program can be obtained by writing the Office of Cancer Communications, National Cancer Institute, Building 31, National Institutes of Health, Bethesda, MD 20014.*

---

* In 1982 the NCI developed a computerized information system to assist physicians nationwide in the selection of a cancer treatment center offering expertise in the treatment of the specific type and stage of cancer for a particular prospective patient. This program is known as PDQ and is available to some 1,800 hospitals and other institutions that have a MEDLARS computer system. If a particular physician does not have access to this computer system, he or she can still get the information by requesting a computer search through an institu-

127

Hospitals that are associated with major university medical schools or research institutes, even if not NCI-affiliated, also usually offer highly qualified senior staff supervision of patient care, availability of scientific and other research staff, adequate laboratories and other facilities, and advanced technology. Many people harbor the notion that because a hospital is "a teaching hospital" they will be treated by book-thumbing medical students or serve as guinea pigs for researchers' latest theories. In fact, standard protocols for patient care are controlled and followed at these hospitals. Senior staff physicians continually supervise and check the skills and thoroughness of care provided by physicians-in-training. And no drug experimentation is done unless it is with an investigational drug approved for patient trials by the FDA, suggested by the supervising physician, and consented to by the patient upon full disclosure of the risks and possible benefits.

As an adult considering a hospital or medical center as your place of treatment, or as a parent concerned with the treatment of your child, you should inquire about the leukemia-treatment protocols that are followed; and assure yourself that a standard, recognized treatment schedule will be followed. Unfortunately, the medical department in charge of leukemia treatment goes by different names in various institutions—such as Leukemia Service, Department of Oncology, Department of Neoplastic Diseases, Department of Hematology, Department of Pediatric Hematology, or Department of Pediatric Oncology.

It is reasonable to expect the diagnosing physician to make the inquiries and gather the information necessary in the choice of a treatment center. He or she can be told of any special requirements, such as geographical area and visitation policies. The physician should also initiate admitting procedures (when a hospital is chosen); and give the patient or patient's family the name of the admitting physician who will at least initially be responsible for treatment. This is particularly important at the very large

---

tion that is hooked up to PDQ. For the name of a nearby PDQ center or for answers to specific questions on the PDQ system, physicians may call NCI's manager of the International Cancer Research Data Bank in Bethesda, Maryland. The telephone number is (301) 496-7403.

medical centers, where admitting procedures can be bewildering. However, it is important to realize that physicians are under no particular obligation regarding referrals, and many will simply recommend the nearest hospital or medical center that has an oncology department. Therefore, the more the patient or family knows about treatment centers, the better.

Patients may be also accepted, free of charge, at the NCI's own clinical center in Bethesda, Maryland. Applications are made by your primary diagnosing physician.

Smaller hospitals and others not associated with the NCI program, or with a university or research institute, may still qualify as an acceptable choice for leukemia patients if they have an active and formal affiliation arrangement with an NCI member institution or university-based hospital. These affiliate hospitals must have at least one key physician trained in leukemia treatment, usually a hematologist who has trained at a leukemia-treatment center.

Such a satellite affiliation is worked out with the parent institution (usually reasonably nearby), which must be assured of the capability of the affiliate's staff, equipment(e.g., blood cell separators), and support services (e.g., nursing, laboratories). Strict supervision is provided by a designated contact at the parent institution. Adherence to the assigned protocol, submission of blood and tissue slides and specimens, and regular transfer of a patient's treatment data and physical and laboratory findings are among the requirements for the affiliate. These satellite hospitals can also participate in the investigative trials of promising new drugs, "pooling" their patient profiles and treatment responses with those of the parent institutions.

This option of getting treatment at an affiliated satellite hospital is suggested primarily for those patients living in an area remote from a major cancer center; or as a recourse for follow-up care, rather than as a choice for induction or relapse treatment.

Less vital aspects of patient life and comfort in the institution are valid considerations, but secondary ones. A person with leukemia, or a parent of a leukemic child, is not likely to be in a state to appraise size of rooms and nursing staff, visiting hours, nearby restaurants and hotels, and considerations such as these.

An important exception is the provision made at the prospective institution for you as a parent of a hospitalized child. You may want to be assured that you can visit your child at any time and remain as long as you wish; and that you can accompany your child for procedures such as X-ray, scans, or marrow extractions. If the institution is not within easy commuting distance, a provision for rooming-in with your child or somewhere else at the hospital can be a significant factor for parents.

Nearby, affordable residences for out-of-town parents of hospitalized children are maintained by some medical centers. Specially designed for this purpose are the Ronald McDonald Houses, not-for-profit residences supported by corporations, local businesses, and individuals. Operated by volunteer boards of directors, Ronald McDonald Houses are located in, or coming to, some sixty cities where medical centers specializing in the treatment of leukemia and other cancers are situated.

MEETING MEDICAL COSTS

Medical costs are a worry for many patients and their families. Those who carry high-option, full coverage health insurance; older persons covered under Medicare; and those of low income who qualify for Medicaid will experience the least strain on personal budget and savings. For middle-income people without all-inclusive health insurance coverage, particularly if the family's main breadwinner is the patient, the financial strain of leukemia treatment can be severe.

The major organizations offering financial assistance are the American Cancer Society and the Leukemia Society of America. Practical household assistance (personnel) is offered by Cancer Care, Inc. The addresses, and type of assistance offered, are listed on pp. 229–34. Your treatment center's social service department can be called on to help arrange these contacts for financial assistance, or even to help file Medicare or Medicaid claims.

For some patients or patients' families, where prolonged and extensive treatment results in medical bills that devastate financial resources, the final recourse has been to declare bankruptcy. This is seen by many people as an extreme solution, and there are serious consequences (such as obtaining credit); but for some families it may seem the only way out. State laws vary on the conditions and provisions for filing personal bankruptcy; and the advice of an attorney should be sought if it is contemplated.

THE SEARCH FOR MEANING AND INFORMATION

Many people when confronted with leukemia go through a period of searching for metaphysical, existential, or religious answers or rationales that will give them some measure of equilibrium. This may involve soul-searching with the objective of reordering priorities; consulting with psychoanalysts and clerics or other spiritual advisers; and reading about or contacting people whose lives have been similarly affected.

This time of crisis, and, for many, time for developing a new approach to life, can be made easier for many parents and patients by exchanges with others in the same situation. There are nationwide organizations for people who are undergoing treatment for cancer and other serious diseases (and for their families), such as Make Today Count, which has over 100 chapters. An organization for parents of young cancer patients is the Candlelighters.

The large medical centers have psychiatric and social service personnel that may be very helpful for those learning to cope with the emotional and practical adjustments that living with leukemia demands. Many of the centers specializing in cancer treatment have ad hoc sessions in which patients and families meet with each other and hospital staff members, including psychological counselors, to discuss feelings, ways of coping, and other information. Some publications resulting from this kind of exchange are listed in "Sources of Help and Information," later in this book.

A number of informative, though brief, pamphlets on leukemia are available from various institutions and health agencies. An excellent and sensitive discussion of leukemia and current treatments, for pre-adolescent youngsters is *You and Leukemia . . . A Day at a Time*, prepared at the Mayo Comprehensive Cancer Center, and available through the W. B. Saunders Publishing Co.

Some patients and parents of leukemic children go on what appears to be an obsessive drive of fact gathering on leukemia and its treatment. Sometimes this is a way of dissipating anger and fear; or of regaining some semblance of control in dealing with the situation. Sometimes it has a more elusive, unconscious motivation: by becoming more like a doctor (informed) one becomes less of a patient (vulnerable). Sometimes fact gathering is a diversion of fear and hostility and is used to challenge the physician or other medical personnel, to catch them in ignorance about some treatment possibility the patient or parent has read or heard about in the news.

It is natural and intelligent for people confronting leukemia in their lives to want to be reasonably well-informed about the disease, about particular treatment procedures, and about research that points to treatment improvements or even cures. You can prepare yourself for conferences with physicians, in which you can ask pointed questions and understand comprehensive answers. Providing this kind of preparation is a primary goal of this book. Becoming more informed can lead to sound decision making, such as in selecting a recognized cancer center instead of a small community hospital as the better place of treatment. It can lead to better understanding of symptoms, and better handling of side effects. It can lead to more truly informed consent to (or dissent from) suggested treatments.

The efforts of informed people have produced a number of services (such as the Ronald McDonald Houses or the Reach to Recovery program for post-mastectomy patients) that benefit other cancer patients and their families. Many national health agencies and research-sponsoring organizations, such as the Leukemia Society of America and the Juvenile Diabetes Foundation, grew from the concern, and organizational and fund-raising initiative of parents of children suffering from these diseases.

Desperation "comparison shopping" for better statistics, new treatments, or a different treatment center most often occurs when the patient or parent mistrusts the physicians, because of perceived or actual indifference; or questions the competence or sensitivity of supporting staff such as nurses or social service workers (although this is less common); or when a relapse occurs, triggering an hysterical search for something better, somewhere.

Persons who feel their physicians don't care about, or have given up on, them or their child, or those with limited intellectual capability and a readiness to accept more positive and simplistic answers, may be lured to quack treatments, such as Laetrile. Such desperation measures will be dealt with later in this chapter.

THE POIGNANCY OF CHILDHOOD LEUKEMIA

The shock and horror that a parent feels on learning that his or her child has leukemia are initially paralyzing. Parents who have been there, and psychologists and others who work with persons suffering the impact of serious—and perhaps fatal— disease diagnosed in their children, say that the paralyzing shock is closely followed by fear and guilt.

The parents feel that something they did or didn't do ("I should have had that sore throat checked by the doctor") allowed leukemia to "happen"; or that their genes are to blame. Some believe that God is punishing them. These agonized parents can be reassured, if not comforted, by the knowledge that nothing they did caused the child's leukemia; and that nothing they could have done would have prevented it.

One of the most difficult emotional hurdles for many parents is the involuntary abdication of their role as the chief protectors of their child, in their own eyes, coupled with the child's realization they are not omnipotent, cannot "make it better" or "make it go away." The young child often feels a loss of faith in, or a betrayal by, the parents; often experiences the illness and hospitalization as a rejection and punishment by the parents, and is likely to feel somehow to blame for what has happened. As one parent said, "We feel ignorant and powerless."

The fear and guilt felt by parents is first expressed as self-blame; this is often followed by rage against others, impotent anger directed at one's spouse, the child's siblings, or the diagnosing physician. Objectivity on the part of hospital staff members is sometimes read as lack of involvement or indifference. This is a source of anger for many parents, and they may lash out at individual nurses, physicians, or other staff members they consider uncaring or even negligent.

These angry parents often seem to believe that anything less than constant and full devotion to the care and cure of their sick child is negligence, a lack of ethics or sympathy, or abandonment. The truth is that no one else can share the intensity of emotional pain, or have the constancy of involvement, that the parent of the leukemic child must bear.

Hospital staff members, to be effective in their care of all patients and to perform their other professional duties, most often cannot "play favorites" or empathize to the degree a parent might secretly wish. The parent has the right, of course, to expect them to be proficient at their work, reasonably communicative, and sensitive to the anguish of the parent as well as of the sick child.

Many parent handbooks prepared by various cancer treatment centers advise that parents set up appointments to meet with the child's primary physician separately, for frank discussion—apart from the physician attentions that involve the child.

What to Tell the Sick Child

Upon diagnosis of leukemia, or during the early days of hospitalization, parents face the wrenching decisions of whether or not to tell the child the truth, and how to explain the disease. The age of the child is a crucial factor in determining how much he or she is told, and in what words; but studies have shown that even those leukemic children not told about the disease come to know its name and implications within the first few months of treatment. Studies and accounts indicate that children feel isolated when they realize that their parents were keeping the truth from them; this also sets up a taboo that prevents the child from expressing many realistic doubts and concerns.

The consensus is that the best policy is for the parent to be frank about the seriousness of the disease, while stressing that good treatment is available. The parent should discuss in detail appropriate to the age of the child the leukemic process, how it differs from normal conditions, and the objectives of treatment.

Those not told, particularly teenagers, are often forced to shoulder another burden: protecting their parents from the greater suffering they assume the parents would feel if they knew the child knew. Psychological studies in this area indicate that a child who is old enough to understand the diagnosis often handles the situation better than the parents; and when the child is presented with information about leukemia and current treatment, he or she becomes less fearful of the disease and more optimistic about the treatment.

The child's reaction to hospitalization varies according to age. Toddlers' anxiety usually appears to be centered on separation from the parent, so the child should be reassured that the parent is coming back and that the "abandonment" is involuntary but necessary. The parent's accompanying the child for procedures such as marrow extractions is also comforting.

Children between four and eight are evidently largely fearful of bodily injury, and can be reassured by explanations of procedures (and also by the presence of the parents during special procedures), and the prospects of normalcy following remission induction.

Older children may want to read about their disease, and to discuss it, and should be encouraged to do so. Studies have shown this information makes them less hostile and more optimistic, and that a fear of dying does not seem to be a significant part of their attitude or behavior. Older children can benefit also from "encounter" or "rap" sessions with other patients of their age group. Youngsters, including teenagers, are very much creatures of today, as one psychologist put it, and not likely to ruminate about death when they have concrete challenges here and now.

"Can this disease kill you?" "Am I going to die?" Studies and experience indicate that this type of direct inquiry is rarely made by children, or if it is, often only once. The best advice seems to be an answer along the lines of: "People have died of leukemia, but many people treated with the drugs like those you're getting are well now, and their disease is under control." And important assurance for younger children would be something like: "You'll be all right because everything that can be done will be done for you; we'll all take care of you."

Relating to the Sick Child

As noted earlier, many children react to their anxiety about hospitalization and their illness with hostility, at least initially. The hostility may be overt, expressed in violent outbursts, rudeness, demands or accusations; or masked by silence, withdrawal, or possibly a defensive posture of removal from the betraying self, the self that got leukemia.

It is important that parents have, or receive help in developing, insights into the child's emotional upheaval, fears, and behavior. Then they can help meet the child's real needs, and not be drawn into exchanges of accusations or forced politeness, or into making tirades, or into a mutual "only the good news" syndrome. It is important also that the child not be avoided because of the parent's own fears—an avoidance which may be perceived by the child as repugnance toward the illness (and the ill child).

The child's forbearance must be respected as the raging is indulged and understood. As Mikie Sherman, in the NIH pamphlet *The Leukemic Child*, expressed her relationship with her hospitalized five-year-old: "I came to welcome Elizabeth's occasional hospital outbursts; to me they represented the breaking of a dam, the sweeping aside of those barriers which she usually maintained at great emotional cost simply so that she would not fall apart. When the barriers broke she was openly recognizing her vulnerability—but in doing so she also became able to receive the love and comfort she needed and which at other times she often rejected."

Many parents also welcome the opportunity to serve the child's physical needs, both in the hospital and at home, in order to feel that they are contributing to the well-being of a child whom they cannot make well. All indications are that this caretaking (bathing, feeding, etc.) is reassuring to children; but parents will hopefully realize that attending to the physical needs of the child does not encompass caring, nor does a limited number of things to "do" for the child render the parent inadequate. To be available in terms of empathy and love; to offer both psychological and practical support; and to discuss, or listen to, the child's fears or concerns, are the invaluable things parents can do for their sick children.

Experts admonish against "spoiling" or overprotecting the sick child. The reasoning is not so much that this breeds an inconsiderate and demanding youngster, but that it encourages a kind of dependency that prevents the child from marshalling his or her own resources to best meet real trials, and undermines the child's self-confidence.

Experts also warn parents not to expect social correctness on the part of the child; or that gifts, visitors, or other overtures will be received gratefully. The parent has to be adult enough to respond to the child's withdrawn or hostile behavior (toward themselves or others) not with hurt or resentment, but with understanding. Experts and parent handbooks suggest that the self-pitying and hostile child can often best be reached by a friendly staff person or, even more likely, a fellow patient of the same age group.

Siblings of the leukemic child, unless they are very young (and even they will realize something is very wrong), should be told honestly of the situation, at whatever explanatory level they can understand. It will be a confusing and frightening time for them. They often feel resentment toward the sick child who has disrupted their own life, and then feel guilty for the resentment.

Siblings should be told the nature of the disease (especially that it is not contagious); reassured that they are healthy (scheduling them for a medical exam may reduce anxiety), and that their anxieties and resentment are normal and acceptable. They may also welcome the opportunity to be of real help to the family. Parents who have reached the coping stage will have to make a special effort to relate to their other children's individual needs.

When the Child Comes Home

Most leukemic children have serious problems when they return home in readjusting to "normal life." Some seek to deny the disease and that they are different from the way they were; some seek a secondary gain through exaggerated helplessness, demands, and abusiveness; many are demanding and fearful, then stoical, by turns. They often feel envious of normal children (even though they may dismiss them as trivial, boring, or immature); and feel that they themselves are tainted and stigmatized. All suffer a severe blow to self-image and self-esteem.

The child in complete remission has no restrictions on activities normal for his or her age; and the child in partial remission can maintain close-to-normal activity levels.

Children on maintenance chemotherapy are most likely receiving drugs that suppress the normal immune response, and exposure to contagious diseases should be avoided. For a school-age child returning to class, this can be difficult to control; but teachers should be asked to contact parents of leukemic children if cases of chicken pox or measles occur in the school. If the white blood cell counts are adequate, most leukemic children can handle other "routine" infections without danger. (Health concerns will be discussed more fully later in the chapter.)

If the protocol included drugs causing hair loss, it usually takes several months following induction chemotherapy for hair to grow back. In the case of toddlers, this may present no special problem. But for older children and teenagers, hair loss may loom as the largest of their immediate concerns.

It is suggested that the parent (with the child's permission) buy a wig as close to the style and color of the child's own hair as possible, first thing—perhaps even before the child comes home from the hospital. Some children may wish to go shopping and select their own wig. (Or they may not want one—remember the "Bald Is Beautiful" boy.)

There is no consensus among patients and parents of leukemic children about whom else to tell, and how much to tell them. Some advocate telling only those who "need" to know—family members and teachers, in the case of a school-age child. Particularly if the child's age-mates are too young for helpful empathy and too ready to taunt away their fears of affliction, it is probably better, according to accounts, not to have the child's condition common knowledge among classmates and friends.

Among those who know the situation either partially or completely, avoidance of the leukemic child and family members as well is an unfortunate occurrence. Mikie Sherman describes the people who withdraw as harboring "an uneasy feeling of being unable to cope or perhaps an unadmitted reaction of repulsion toward the ill or handicapped. They have perhaps only internalized more than others some of the prevailing attitudes of our society:

that illness is an unpleasant deviance . . . and that the ill are some-how themselves responsible for their unlucky fate."

And yet of course some friends remain committed, and, if any-thing, more caring and helpful than before. Most patient and parent accounts of their adjustments describe significant support and empathy by a number of family members and friends, and sometimes by acquaintances who surprisingly offer themselves in time of need.

Attention to the Child's Health

The leukemic child at home will most likely be scheduled for frequent blood tests (usually weekly or biweekly), which can be done by the family physician or the child's pediatrician, at a local medical facility or at the leukemia treatment center's follow-up clinic, if it is reasonably nearby. Whatever the arrangement, close contact between the follow-up physician and the child's leukemia-center physician must be established.

The child must take maintenance medication regularly, often daily. He or she will be scheduled for regular medical check-ups, blood counts and chemistries, and marrow tests at the leukemia treatment center or a designated facility. Courses of reinforcement therapy may be scheduled every month or few months.

Parents are advised to keep a medication-schedule calendar that includes the dates for tests and check-ups, and to keep their own records of clinic visits (blood counts, treatment given). It's sug-gested that a parent also keep brief records of the child's general health, dating any unexplained symptoms, fever, or side effects of medication. These records can be important for informing the clinic physician during check-ups, or if illness develops between clinic visits.

Many parents find that the leukemic child adopts a level of activity that he or she can handle; and that rarely do they pursue or initiate activity beyond their capabilities (it's too frustrating). A good diet is advisable; light, nutritious snacks may be more favorably received than large, heavy meals. Multivitamins can be given. Constipation can be countered with foods that contain a lot of roughage—fruits, vegetables, bran flakes, and whole grain breads; or the physician may suggest a laxative or enema. Nausea and vomiting can be controlled by medication, and can sometimes be reduced by avoiding sweets, including sweetened beverages, and fried or fatty foods. Sore mouth can be alleviated by a mouthwash; both can be prescribed by the physician. If the maintenance medication includes prednisone, there may be heartburn or peptic distress (countered by a glass of milk or an antacid with each dose), and weight gain (countered by a limit on fatty food, salt seasoning, and salty snacks).

Tylenol or other nonaspirin analgesics (generic name: acetaminophen) may be given for aches, pains, and minor infections.

All tablets, including maintenance medication, vitamins, and analgesics, can be crushed and mixed with applesauce, banana, custard, and the like.

As noted in chapter 3, herpes viruses can be hazardous to the patient on medication that diminishes the immune response; however, new drugs have been developed against chicken pox and herpes simplex virus (most often manifest in children as cold sores). Immunization (against chicken pox) or preventive medication (against herpes simplex) may be advised by the physician. If the child is exposed to chicken pox or develops cold sores, the physician should be notified.

Live virus vaccines (regular measles, German measles or rubella, mumps, polio) should not be given to leukemia patients. Family physicians and pediatricians will likely know this but adamant school officials may need a note from the child's physician. Diphtheria, whooping cough, and tetanus immunizations are not live vaccines and are safe.

Many patients are anxious about possible signs of an approaching relapse—that they may miss telltale signs or symptoms. They can be reassured that the frequent blood tests and the regular marrow tests will show evidence if a relapse is imminent—either through the presence of blasts (immature cells) in the blood or marrow, or through abnormal numbers or proportions of blood or marrow components.

Several of the most important blood studies, and normal values per milliliter of sample for these tests in children are: hemoglobin (red cell substance that carries oxygen)—eleven to fourteen grams; number of white blood cells—4,000 to 11,000; number of blood platelets—150,000 to 350,000.

These values are calculated as percentages or actual amounts within a given blood-sample volume. Many people deviate—run consistently higher or lower—from normal values and are not ill. Maintenance medication, infections, conditions producing anemia, and other causes unrelated to leukemia may distort the blood-sample picture. A bone marrow study must be done to confirm whether or not there has been a recurrence of leukemia.

If any of the following symptoms—which are the same as the initial symptoms of leukemia—do occur between regularly scheduled check-ups, the physician should be contacted: easy bruising or blood splotches under the skin; any abnormal bleeding; marked tiredness, breathlessness, or pallor; bone or joint pain; fever without apparent infection; night sweats; swelling of the gums; and swollen lymph nodes. Other symptoms that should prompt a call to the doctor include rashes of any kind; severe constipation or diarrhea; and any pain of unusual intensity, including headache.

All parents and patients hope that their children or they will be the ones to achieve a cure. The first relapse, if it occurs, is apt to be as devastating as the initial diagnosis. Parents quoted in the American Cancer Society's *Parents' Handbook on Leukemia* (1978) say: "We seek the best treatment possible and hope that new drugs will be found for use if further relapses occur. Hope seems to be a necessary component for living and not a disavowal of the fact that death is inevitable for everyone. At least we can learn not to wait to share ourselves, our talents and emotions, until the right or convenient time."

THE ADULT WITH LEUKEMIA

No experience of his life, wrote the political columnist Stewart Alsop, was "more mixed up than the peculiar hell-to-heaven-to-purgatory existence I have had since I was first diagnosed as an acute leukemic. In a way no experience has been more interesting than living in intermittent intimacy with the gentleman I have come to think of as Uncle Thanatos, and sometimes, when I have been feeling very sick, as dear old Uncle Thanatos."

Mr. Alsop, who died of leukemia in 1974, at age sixty, took an intense interest in leukemia research and treatment, and took a clinical as well as a subjective interest in his own case and its vagaries. He described in his 1973 book *Stay of Execution* (Harper & Row) his feelings, memories, life-style, handicaps, pleasures, and insights over a two-year period as he experienced the ordeal of leukemia.

Mr. Alsop's eloquent book, which steers rigorously away from self-pity, gives the reader a firsthand battle account. Alluding seldom to bouts with despair, Mr. Alsop is nonetheless able to speak of his periods of depression, when "there was the temptation to let things slide, to say the hell with it." He speaks of periods of euphoria and gratitude, and of the lurking fear:

"It was always present, like a kind of background music. Sometimes it receded almost into inaudibility; and then sometimes it would come blaring back, accompanied by a sense of incredulity. 'My God, I really do have cancer, and I really am going to die.'

"The fear leaps out, every fourth page or so, from my notebooks . . ."

He was astonished to discover that a fellow patient (at NCI's clinical center), a woman in remission who came to the hospital for maintenance therapy, was "quite obviously telling the simple truth" when she denied worrying about a relapse, saying she was too busy with her children and never thought about it except when she came for her tests.

The most looming pragmatic fear that Mr. Alsop had was the possibility of having to endure being placed in an isolation room. Another personal priority: he insisted that his physician enter into his chart a prescription for martinis before dinner, in case he might have to be hospitalized when this physician was away or unavailable.

Priorities, whether among fears, joys, or simple pleasures, vary a great deal among the adults recounting their experiences as leukemia victims. Undoubtedly this is because they can be leukemia victims only part time, and are themselves the rest of the time.

Angela Ambrosia, who had been under treatment for leukemia since she was sixteen, wrote, as a married woman in her mid-twenties: "To this day, I can't get over staying out late and not having to answer to anyone—just having fun with my husband . . . the feeling I have of still being on my honeymoon . . . no longer being afraid of the dark."

Kelly Sveinson, a Canadian patient who makes his living in advertising and describes himself as a successful public speaker, stays true to form in his book *Learning to Live with Cancer*. He has an almost Norman Vincent Peale approach toward positive thinking, full of advice on adopting attitudes and objectives.

This optimistic, "willpower" approach might be just the sort of guidance desired by some patients. Others may choose a more hedonistic, existential, religious, or even nihilistic route for themselves. Many patients strive to continue their work, careers, or roles much as before; others surprise themselves by choosing a totally different life-style or set of interests.

Patients admit that incorporating pain, medical treatments, frustrations, "temporariness," fear, and sometimes despair into one's life is an awesome and often awful process. But most of them attest that it need not be overwhelming, at least not all the time.

The need for other people, the need to keep one's spirit intact, and the persistence of hope seem to be universal.

Besides the issue of whom and how much to tell about one's illness, finances are primary concerns of adult leukemia patients, particularly those in the work force. One is treated differently in the office. One can work only part time. Another must claim disability payments. A male patient's wife must get a job; his son will have to take over many of his duties. One woman is promoted "upstairs" and given nothing to do; her smallest accomplishments are greeted with exaggerated praise.

Illness may also raise domestic issues. Problems with sex may arise. Should the house be sold? Children may seem fearful or condescending or overly solicitous.

These, and undoubtedly many other problems, will beset the adult leukemia patient. Being able to reach out to others, as well as finding new strengths in oneself, appear to be among the silver linings of leukemia for those who write or tell about it. As Stewart Alsop wrote, "One compensation for getting really sick is the repeated discovery that people are nicer than they seem to be."

Handling the Side Effects of Therapy

Most of the nonhazardous side effects resulting from chemo-therapy are the same for adults as for children, and were discussed earlier in this chapter. There are two additions: diarrhea may occur with some of the adult medications, and can be controlled with prescribed drugs; and cystitis—pain with urination, blood in urine—may occur when under treatment with cyclo-phosphamide, and can be controlled with large fluid intake and prescribed medication, if necessary.

For sore mouth, some patients advise gargling with a glass of lukewarm water with salt dissolved in it. Taken about ten minutes before eating, it can boost food intake.

As for loss of appetite, patient advice is wildly varying. A young man finds beer and pretzels always appealing when nothing else is. A young woman found eating Chinese food with chopsticks just her speed. A hospitalized older man found that a picnic-type meal, with napkins, silverware, and wine glasses from home, made his day. Another older man discovered chocolate ice cream on a stick hit the spot.

Ameliorating Drugs

There are numerous nonprescription and prescription drugs to relieve physical or psychological suffering—analgesics, tranquilizers, mood elevators, sedatives—that may be requested by the patient or suggested by the physician. This is an area of considerable controversy.

At one extreme, the antimedication adherents, whose position is only rarely based on stiff-upper-lip morality, contend that obliterating patients' distress often also obliterates their personality; that the drugs induce dependency that infantalizes patients and prevents them from making real choices and decisions. The promedication advocates contend that a cancer patient has enough to deal with, and that struggling to cope with physical pain and psychic distress is enervating, consuming, and counterproductive to battling for one's life in a meaningful way.

Of course there is no correct position on the issue of someone else's pain or debilitation. Consultation with the physician and with a psychologist or psychoanalyst may help the patient formulate a policy on drug relief for the present and future, after declaring his or her intentions—to live as drug-free as tolerable, for example, or to minimize suffering above all.

It is not rare for hospitals to give patients analgesics and sedatives routinely; and instances of psychoactive drugs being administered without the patient's, or patient's family's, knowledge do occur. The husband of one patient was increasingly dismayed to find his wife placid and uncomprehending; he was told she was being given "happy pills." Not only were the nurses patronizing in their description of the medication; the husband discovered the pills were phenothiazine, an antipsychotic drug that renders patients "manageable." The patient or a family member has the right to inquire about the name and nature of any drug being administered and to refuse it, if so desired.

It is estimated by the National Cancer Institute that 30 percent of cancer patients suffer severe pain and require drugs for relief; NCI surveys indicate that morphine and other narcotics control pain for over 90 percent of these patients. Clinical tests comparing injectable heroin to morphine found it no more effective; but since heroin is easier to dissolve (requiring less volume of solution), it may be preferable for patients with wasted muscles or those who require large amounts of the drug.

In 1981, the NCI reported that evaluations of marijuana over a five-year period showed convincing evidence of the drug's effectiveness for many patients in controlling nausea and vomiting due to chemotherapy. It has been recognized also as a pain suppressant and mood elevator. It is estimated that some 50,000 cancer patients each year begin chemotherapy and suffer severe nausea and vomiting—in some cases to the degree that they ask to have chemotherapy stopped. The NCI is, therefore, making a marijuana derivative available to medical centers whose pharmacies have a Schedule I license, which ensures precautions in handling and dispensing drugs the FDA believes to have a high potential for abuse. The marijuana is available to cancer patients as capsules containing the active ingredient known as THC (tetrahydrocannabinol).

Stoicism, on the part of a person whose life is seriously threatened by illness, is not always a voluntary posture, especially for the patient who has not had the opportunity to discuss drug relief of distress. Sometimes patients refuse drugs because they imagine the medicine will induce a zombie-like state that might disappoint family or friends, or destroy their self-image.

The question of the possible use of any prescription analgesics, sedatives, or psychoactive drugs; as well as their effectiveness; their common or unusual side effects; and any dangers as to their use in combination with other drugs may be broached to the physician freely by the patient or a family member.

Some patients seem to fear their own anticipated fear above all. They are afraid that they will be overwhelmingly terrified at some possible future stage in their illness when they won't be able to handle their fear or pain. This thought is particularly likely to plague the "proud," the stoical, or the seemingly resigned patient, who fear as readily as anyone else but have a tremendous investment in not expressing it.

Any discussion with the physician on the use of ameliorating drugs should, of course, be limited to drug usage within the boundaries of acceptable medical practice.

Psychotherapy

According to a 1982 report in *The New England Journal of Medicine*, as many as one-fourth of all patients who experience abdominal-distress *reactions* to actual drug administrations learn to psychologically "turn on" symptoms of nausea and vomiting in *anticipation* of their next treatment. Desensitization techniques commonly used to overcome phobias are being tried to reduce or eliminate this psychosomatic illness—with good results, according to the article. The technique involves inducing a state of deep muscular relaxation in patients, then guiding them verbally—they will later do it mentally themselves—over each distressful sensation while persuading them to dispel it. This technique is suggested also to help negate the actual, as well as the anticipated, side effects of chemothreapy.

DESPERATION "CURES" AND THERAPIES

In the 1950s, a substance called Krebiozen was widely publicized as a painless cure for cancer. You don't hear anything about it today, although it has a niche in the history of popularized remedies for cancer—remedies that cling to the fringes of medicine for a time, then disappear as their promises fail and their promoters fade. Simple yet magical cures for cancer have been around for a long time. While peering nearsightedly at rings in a jewelry store recently, one of us (Cynthia Margolies) was approached by a clerk who confidently recommended that a mixture of cucumbers, carrots, and parsley, consumed daily, would not only restore perfect sight, but would even cure cancer. This kind of advice is probably relatively harmless, but when there is an organized promotion of a specific product that is refused acknowledgment by the mainstream of the medical profession, the touted substance is often one that falls under "unproven methods of cancer management," or, less formally, "cancer quackery." The most recent "potion" to attract notoriety, or celebrity, depending on how you look at it, is Laetrile.

Laetrile (common chemical name, amygdalin) is not a mysterious substance, but a naturally occurring plant product found in the kernels of bitter almonds and apricots. It was "rediscovered" in the late 1950s, and later received a mounting promotion as a cancer cure, primarily by a group of advocates in California, who now call Laetrile a vitamin and cancer a deficiency disease;* the group includes several physicians who dispense Laetrile in their practices.

Over the last twenty years, Laetrile has been biochemically analyzed for a possible mode of action against cancer cells, and has been tested in animals to assess any anti-cancer activity in various investigations made by the National Cancer Institute (NCI) and under NCI research contracts at other cancer research centers. None of these tests demonstrated any evidence that

* G. Edward Griffin, "World Without Cancer," transcript of film narration, from American Media, Westlake Village, Ca. (undated); also in *Laetrile Case Histories: The Richardson Cancer Clinic Experience* (New York: Bantam Books, Inc., 1977), pp. 5–6.

Laetrile benefited animals with tumors; and no drug has been proved active in human cancer which does not show anti-cancer activity in experimental animals. For this reason, Laetrile was never scheduled for trials in humans.

However, in the 1970s there arose a public and political uproar around Laetrile, with promoters claiming that the marketplace should be the judge—that is, people should be allowed to buy or be given Laetrile treatment if they wanted (twenty-three states have legalized Laetrile, despite a continuing ban by the Federal Food and Drug Administration (FDA) on its interstate distribution). Laetrile advocates claim also that there is a conspiracy of the medical establishment and petroleum and pharmaceutical companies to prevent the widespread use of Laetrile.*

In response, the NCI sponsored a study in 1980 to determine possible toxic effects of Laetrile, which involved a small group of cancer patients at the Mayo Clinic in Rochester, Minnesota; this was followed by an NCI-sponsored trial of Laetrile in 156 cancer patients at four cancer research centers. The institutions were the Mayo Clinic; UCLA Jonsson Comprehensive Cancer Center, Los Angeles; Memorial Sloan-Kettering Cancer Center, New York City; and the University of Arizona Health Sciences Center, Tucson. All enrolled patients gave informed consent to the treatments; the patients were those for whom no other treatment had been effective, or those for whom no proven treatment existed and who chose Laetrile over other investigational drugs. One-third of the patient group had no prior chemotherapy. Patients received "metabolic therapy" as advocated by Laetrile practitioners, which consists of a diet that favors fresh fruits, vegetables, and whole grains, prohibits animal products, includes pancreatic enzymes and large doses of vitamins A, C, and E and moderate amounts of B-complex vitamins and minerals. (This regimen is sometimes referred to as "holistic therapy" or "orthomolecular medicine" by advocates.)

Results of the clinical trial were reported by Charles Moertel,

---

* John A. Richardson, M.D., and Patricia Griffin, R.N., *Laetrile Case Histories*, pp. 97–102; see also Richard D. Lyons, "Backers of Laetrile Charge a Plot Is Preventing the Cure of Cancer," *The New York Times*, 13 July 1977.

M.D., chairman of the Department of Oncology, Mayo Clinic, at the annual meeting of the American Society of Clinical Oncology, in Washington, D.C., on April 30, 1981. A summary of the investigators' reports, prepared for the nation's news media, began:

"The purpose of the trial, which began in July 1980, was to determine in a scientific study whether Laetrile plus a 'metabolic therapy' program of special diet, enzymes, and vitamins, did or did not have anti-tumor activity. According to results of the study: no substantive benefit from Laetrile has been observed in terms of cure, improvement, or slowing the advance of the cancer, improvement of symptoms related to cancer, or extension of lifespan."

At the end of his slide presentation to the meeting, Dr. Moertel concluded:

> *We fully realized as we began this study that if we achieved negative results, this would not be convincing to the Laetrile zealots, but it was not our intention to convince the zealots. We do hope, however, that these results will be helpful to thoughtful cancer patients and their families as they consider therapeutic alternatives. Heretofore they have been badly confused. We also hope these results will be helpful to the physician as he counsels his cancer patients. Laetrile has been tested; it is not effective.*

James F. Holland, M.D., chairman of the Department of Neoplastic Diseases at New York City's Mount Sinai Medical Center, sounded a pragmatic note in filing an affidavit in 1977 supporting the FDA's continued ban on Laetrile, following his eight months' exchange-scientist work in Soviet cancer hospitals:

> *There is no private enterprise in the Soviet Union, and drugs are manufactured or imported and distributed for cancer, based upon demonstrated activity . . . Laetrile is neither manufactured, imported or distributed in the Soviet Union. It is important to recognize that this is an additional way of putting the lie to the innuendo that American medicine is profiteering by keeping effective cancer drugs from cancer patients. That accusation fails of its own weight. It is also rele-*

> *vant that the Soviet Union, the world's second richest*
> *and second most powerful nation, a country well-known*
> *in the past for adopting ideas and chemical formulae*
> *without paying royalties, has not seen fit to appropriate*
> *Laetrile. Perhaps, they recognize it as worthless. An*
> *old Russian proverb would put it, "one doesn't steal an*
> *empty sack."*

It is easy to be angry at the unorthodox practitioners and just as easy to understand their motivations: for most it's money—in addition to their ministrations they sell their prescriptions, which is not done by reputable physicians; for some it's vindication against a society or profession which has neglected them or refused to honor their talents; and for a few it may indeed be a misguided if grandiose belief that their methods or products will work where the efforts of organized medicine have failed.

It is almost impossible to be angry with desperate cancer patients who turn to unorthodox therapies, or even with family members or friends who urge it because of their own anxious need to recommend *something* that seems more promising, or less frightening. Here the motivations are more complicated. The "freedom of choice" banner being waved by Laetrile promoters flatters our sense of exercising "rights." But this area—the type of medical treatment to select—is in fact one where most of us rely on the guidance of medical experts.

Why, in fact, do people "choose" Laetrile? Among the lures of Laetrile are that it's "natural" and noninvasive, as opposed to conventional treatments that are often painful, accompanied by unpleasant side effects, and sometimes physically disfiguring. There is also the lure of the easy answer that will put "big medicine" in its place—along with big government and big bucks. And, as Oliver Wendell Holmes said in 1842: "There is a class of minds much more ready to believe that which is at first sight incredible, and because it is incredible, than what is generally thought reasonable." Also, Laetrile proponents propagandize extensively, and aggressively solicit prospective clients, sometimes phoning diagnosed cancer patients, visiting them at home, inviting them to lectures, films "documenting" Laetrile's benefits, and so on. Orville Kelly of Burlington, Iowa, the founder of Make Today Count (see "Sources of Help and Information," later in this book), reports that from the day his aid organization for cancer patients was announced in the media, "The pressure upon me as a cancer patient and upon my wife . . . to begin Laetrile therapy . . . has never stopped. [Callers and writers would contend that] chemotherapy drugs were poison and were killing me."

Of all the tragedies associated with Laetrile use, the most awful must be the case in which patients forego conventional treatment when their disease has the potential for control, turn to Laetrile therapy, then return to reputable doctors when it is too late, when their disease has metastasized or overwhelmed vital organs. Many physicians cite this danger in rejecting the opinion that Laetrile is harmless even if ineffective; it creates a climate of acceptance that encourages people to believe "there must be something to it." Dr. William A. Nolen describes such cases in his book about his investigations of miracle cures, *Healing: A Doctor in Search of a Miracle* (New York: Random House, 1974).

Should the government step aside and allow the marketplace to function with regard to health products and medical treatment? Should the 1962 amendments to the Food, Drug and Cosmetic Act be revoked, so that drugs need not be proven effective for their intended use? Or, rather, doesn't the public have the right to protection in an area such as medical treatment, where they cannot have sufficient knowledge to protect themselves against quackery and poor practice?

This is what the licensing of physicians is about, why we have drug standards and restrictions, why there are accreditation standards for hospitals. A patient can refuse treatment, can seek another professional opinion, can volunteer for experimental treatment. But a patient has the right to be protected—to know that he or she is dealing with qualified professionals and institutions, that drugs which may be used are those that have been approved and shown to be beneficial according to rigorous trial criteria.

Studies among patients who opt for Laetrile as compared to those who seek "establishment" care turn up one significant difference: the Laetrile group had a much higher percentage of persons who felt their doctors had abandoned them, medically and emotionally.

Dr. Glen Davidson, professor of psychiatry at Southern Illinois

University School of Medicine, has made a special study of cancer patients and their families. He feels the emphasis is wrong when hopes are placed solely on cure and the physician's abilities, rather than on coping and the patient's abilities. When the physician can no longer promise effective help, the patient feels abandoned and panicked.

Other studies have shown that most seriously ill patients are able to cope with their situation if they are encouraged to do so, rather than being manipulated and infantalized by others.

CHAPTER FIVE

RESEARCH DIRECTIONS

Early in 1982, the American Cancer Society launched a six-year research project that will attempt to answer why some people get cancer and others don't. More than one million Americans will be asked to complete questionnaires covering some 500 pieces of personal information that may have a bearing on cancer causation, under topics such as diet, occupation, and use of drugs. The survey is biased toward older persons, since incidence of cancer increases with advancing age. Volunteer surveyors will follow up survey subjects in 1984, 1986, and 1988 to record any changes in health.

This mass epidemiological study will attempt to isolate statistically significant personal characteristics and habits, and environmental exposures or situations that may correlate with either good health or susceptibility to cancer. If cases of cancer or cancer deaths occur among survey subjects, those subjects' questionnaires will be searched for common links to the development of cancer.

This project is aimed at achieving a base of hard data that can be used predictively. Until now, most epidemiological surveys related to cancer have been done only after researchers have been hit over the head with data implicating a cancer link far too strong to be coincidental—such as the data on cigarette smoking, or working with asbestos. The hoped-for predictive possibilities that might come from the new survey's data could be used, for example, to alert cancer-susceptible individuals to the need for frequent medical examinations, specific tests, or advisable preventive treatment or life-style changes. The project's data will hopefully develop various profiles of cancer-susceptible individuals, ranging from "unlikely" to "very likely" for the development of cancer.

Smaller-scale research efforts to develop indicators of cancer susceptibility were discussed in chapter 2. Examples given included the testing of the cells of persons from "cancer families" for DNA mutation following exposure to low levels of radiation or chemical carcinogens, and analyzing metabolic products of tobacco-smoke carcinogens as to what effect they have on a given smoker's cell samples (whether they produce a potent end product that can bind to DNA and cause mutation, thus flagging a high-risk individual).

As noted in chapter 2, only three types of cancer are directly associated with specific inheritable genetic abnormalities—two types of kidney cancer and a tumor of the eye's retina. Although there are genetic markers in the cells of some leukemia patients— e.g., the "Philadelphia chromosome" of chronic myelocytic leukemia or the large quantities of a particular MHC antigen on cells of acute lymphocytic leukemia patients—these markers are seen after disease diagnosis and may be consequential to leukemia rather than causally related. About half of all leukemia patients fail to exhibit detectable genetic abnormalities.

A number of types of cancer can now be ferreted out by the appearance of malignancy-associated markers (e.g., the presence of "fetal" proteins) on cells, in the blood, in the urine, or in specific tissues or secretions, before the disease is prevalent enough for standard diagnostic methods. This is particularly helpful for individuals who are at high risk for a particular type of cancer, such as members of "cancer families," or for cancer patients in remission, who can be checked for residual or recurrent disease.

Possible residual or recurrent leukemia in patients in remission cannot presently be reliably detected by other than cautionary signs (e.g., CNS symptoms, abnormal proportions of the various blood cell types, low platelet counts) in the absence of abnormal cells or cell proportions in the bone marrow. As noted earlier, a possible relapse is indicated by marrow analysis weeks or months sooner than would be apparent by blood samples alone. However the presence in the blood of a particular enzyme, called deoxynucleotidyl transferase, or its presence in lymphocyte samples, is now believed by many researchers to be linked to residual leukemia; and at high levels, it is linked—or at least strongly associated—with imminent relapse. Tests to check for the enzyme have been developed; and its diagnostic value is being analyzed. Another possible associate in leukemia development is a virus-like particle containing enzyme activity (the enzyme is reverse transcriptase) that allows RNA viruses to form DNA; the particle has been found in the cells of virtually every patient with acute leukemia tested for it. However, *infectivity* of the particle has not been demonstrated; and it is unclear whether this is a marker for leukemia or just a coincidental and latent viral presence.

One of the major problems that leukemia researchers are tackling is the lack of leukemia-specific cellular antigens, or other specific attributes or lacks—markers that could target leukemic cells for customized drugs that would starve, paralyze, or directly kill them. With the exception of the drug asparaginase, which exploits a metabolic lack specific to leukemic cells, anti-leukemic drugs demonstrate preferences for cycle-active cells, for cells especially responsive to hormone-type drugs, and even for white blood cells in particular; all of which make the drugs useful against leukemic cells, but not exclusive to them.

One of the distressing points made in the recent studies of natural "cancer genes" in humans is that the guilty genes seem to make a normal, human cellular protein that may be abnormal only in amount, time, or place (i.e., cell type) of appearance. Since many normal cells evidently make small amounts of the same proteins, fashioning an antagonist to the protein would create a drug no more specific than many of those in use today. The diagnosis-linked enzymes mentioned above suffer the same drawback of nonspecificity for purposes of targeting drugs.

However, researchers are becoming much more intimate with leukemic cells and the events that accompany a cell's transformation to a leukemic one; they will find ways to interfere with, or correct, that genetic programming. There are a number of new approaches to eliminating the leukemic cell currently being explored, and this chapter will discuss some of them.

In the meantime, treatment efforts must focus on leukemic-cell destruction—preferentially, if not exclusively; revitalization of normal bone marrow activity; bolstering of immune-response mechanisms; and overcompensation for immune-system lacks. Successful arrest, or even partial remission, of leukemia offers a potential for cure.

Work continues at several leukemia treatment centers to develop reliable prognostic indicators for patients—those significant personal factors that can help predict response to chemotherapy. This work was outlined in chapter 3, and is further discussed in this chapter under "Tailoring Chemotherapy and Patient Prognosis." The approach allows a treatment schedule that is customized, and gives the patient, the patient's family, and the attending physician a clearer idea of the probable outcome of treatment.

Leukemia research moves forward on many fronts, from studies centered on details of cellular life (normal versus leukemic) to refinements in marrow transplantation and the fine-tuning of chemotherapy use. In this chapter's overview of research activity, the first distinction that should be made is between the major research categories, *basic* and *clinical*.

Basic research in biomedical science involves the study of anatomy and physiology in the microscopic world; investigators observe, theorize, test their theories, and build from earlier research findings. Their work is centered on the activities and responses of living cells or certain aspects or components of cellular life. A handful of facts can put their work in perspective for the rest of us: in a drop of blood as big as the printed dot on this i, there are about 5 million red cells, 300,000 platelets, and 7,000 white cells; the average cell has about a million proteins including about 3,000 different kinds of enzymes, and is orchestrating some 20,000 reactions at any given instant; a cell's DNA, if it were stretched out with all genes end-to-end, rather than packed into the cell's nucleus, would be six feet in length.

Basic research is usually conducted in the laboratory with cells or cellular components "under glass" (what used to be called test-tube studies) or through animal studies measuring responses to therapeutic innovations. The work is often exploratory and long-term, and findings may not be applicable to patient care for years. Dr. Walter Gilbert, Nobel Prize-winning chemist of Harvard University, said, in accepting his 1980 Prize: "The cutting edge of science is basic research; and what we learn in basic research we can later apply." The main areas of basic research relevant to leukemia today are genetics, immunology, virology, pharmacology, cellular kinetics (i.e., movements and changes), and the catchall, cell biology.

What people hear or read about in the news as "breakthroughs" in medicine are applications to patients of experimental methods or substances—applications that came from basic research and probably had a long gestation there; and such advances belong to the category of clinical research. Clinical research involves bringing a technique out of the lab to the "clinic" for use on patients on an experimental basis. Patient trials are preceded by carefully documented preliminary studies (such as with cultured cells and groups of animals) that produce evidence of probable beneficial results for patients.

When a new treatment is brought into patient use, it is considered investigational, often for a period of years. When dealing with toxic drugs or invasive treatments such as irradiation or surgery, risk factors and compromise of bodily integrity must be closely weighed against probable benefit. In the case of medical technology involving little or no conceivable bodily harm to the patient, such as computerized scanning, ultrasound diagnosis, or flow cytofluorometry (in which only cell samples are examined), research is only hampered by the time, talent, and money needed for refinement and accuracy.

The investigational period is needed to determine such things as: what categories of patients benefit, or don't benefit, from a given treatment; consistency of results among patients with similar medical profiles; base lines for interpretation and comparison of patient readings or findings (What is a normal brain scan? In what ways is the patient's scan abnormal? What do the abnormalities indicate?); and serious immediate, or long-term, side effects. This kind of data can be accumulated only through studies of, and results from, a series of people over a period of time.

In the case of drug usage, the federal Food and Drug Administration requires standard testing procedures. Since 1962, the FDA has been empowered to set criteria for bringing out any new drug, ensuring that drugs are not only safe, but effective for their intended use. The drugs, whether given for diagnostic or treatment purposes, must give evidence of probable benefit; the safe-dosage range must be established; and side effects must be published.

In general, new drugs are tested on animals for a number of years to check for effectiveness as well as toxicity (i.e., dangerous effects on nontarget tissues or organs). Then, assuming a drug passes animal testing, it enters a three-phase protocol of testing in humans, which is carried out over a period of years.

In the first phase, the drug is given to a small number of healthy volunteers, in small amounts, to determine the method of administration (e.g., oral or intravenous); any toxic effects; and a probable safe-dosage range. In the second phase, the drug is tried on a number of people who have the disease the drug is intended to eradicate or alleviate. If testing indicates benefit (e.g., in the case of cancer, if tumors shrink, or blood tests give readings closer to normal) and no unwarranted harm, the trials continue.

Phase three involves extensive testing of a drug's effectiveness in treating a specific condition or disease in a large number of people—from several hundred to several thousand. It is evaluated as the single medication for some patients, and in combination with other appropriate drugs for other groups of patients—to check for advantageous or dangerous combined effects. Phase three tests continue to assess the drug's safety—especially any delayed side effects—and optimal dosages for various patient categories are determined (e.g., children, the elderly, those with heart disease). The drug sponsor, which may be a chemical company, a research institute or, often, a pharmaceutical company, then submits its data to the FDA and requests marketing approval.

If a new drug application is approved, manufacture and distribution may proceed. The manufacturer must report to the FDA every three months during the first year (on such things as adverse effects when combined with other drugs, or side effects that may arise with long-term use), every six months in the second year, and once a year thereafter.

The main areas of clinical research relevant to leukemia today are immunotherapy, bone marrow transplantation, testing new anti-leukemia drugs, customizing supportive therapy, and tailoring treatment protocols to the individual patient profile.

GENETICS

The concepts of classical genetics—which explain the reappearance of identical traits from one generation to another and also account for trait variation—were formulated in the mid-nineteenth century by the Austrian monk Gregor Mendel. Studying generations of sweet-pea plants and experimenting with cross-fertilizations among the plants, Mendel came to the conclusion that something called genes were the medium and the message of inheritable characteristics.

Basing his work on observable traits (such as seed color of the sweet peas), Mendel, reasoning inductively, hypothesized two genes governing each trait, one from each parent, to allow for expected characteristics (identical genes = homozygous offspring) and diverse possibilities (different genes = heterozygous offspring). The trait *exhibited* by offspring of heterozygotes could be explained by the theory of dominant and recessive genes (see Glossary, "Mendel's Law").

His principles were generally proven correct, although they could not anticipate linked genes, or gene rearrangements that occur naturally prior to chromosome division at fertilization. (Linked genes are those that must be "turned on" simultaneously or in concert with others to produce a particular protein, or to act as an effective "tollbooth" (or permissive signal) for DNA activity. Gene rearrangements occur as nearby nucleotide groups sometimes change places.)

It would be a hundred years before the scientific world became acquainted with the stuff of which genes are made. Genetic understanding has been revolutionized within the last fifty years, from the vague concepts of inheritance based on observable traits (e.g., eye color, hair color) to the exploration and analysis of DNA itself.

The large majority of current genetic studies are at the level of basic research. Scientists have analyzed and mapped less than 1 percent of human genetic material—that is, they know what these genes do and how they are composed, and where on the chromosomes they are located. Most of this work has involved the presence of presumed genetic errors: the cells of members of a family

159

which suffer from a hereditary disease are searched for DNA abnormalities that are fairly obvious under the microscope, or obvious when the suspect DNA segment is matched with presumably normal DNA. With the new technologies of gene-splicing, to be discussed in the next section, and nucleotide sequencing, much smaller degrees of abnormalities will be detectable much more quickly.

Besides the piece-by-piece analysis of abnormal genes that are derived from mutations and linked to human diseases, and the mapping of such genes, basic genetic research particularly directed to malignancy includes: (1) investigations concerning oncogenes, both those that are virus-derived and productive of animal cancers, and the native, counterpart human genes that normally lie dormant; (2) studies of regulatory genes that control apparent oncogenes, including work on how these regulatory genes are "turned on" or bypassed in the malignant transformation of a cell; (3) work concerning DNA mutations and rearrangements and the normal repair process; (4) studies of the powerful effects that can be generated by very small changes in DNA coding; (5) studies of the activities and awesome influence of the unit of genes that constitutes the major histocompatibility complex, which appears to determine the stringency and vigor of an individual's entire immune-response system; and (6) investigations related to gene splicing, using microorganisms to churn out cancer-combative human proteins.

Work in the first five areas listed above has been outlined or discussed elsewhere in this book. In this section, the new technology of gene splicing, or genetic engineering, will be described. This technology holds the potential for mass production of medically useful human substances to be used for individuals who lack them; and, eventually, for inserting genetic repairs or replacements into human cells.

Genetic Engineering

In recent years, genetic research and the prospects of new life forms being created in laboratories have received much media attention, conjuring up in many minds mixtures of fear and hope.

Central to these issues are the deciphering of the genetic code and the innovations of gene manipulation, known as genetic engineering. The rapid advances in genetic engineering (which includes cell fusions as well as gene splicing) are being applied to create healthier plants and animals, as well as to provide supplements for promoting healthier humans. The focus here will be on gene splicing—also known as recombinant DNA technology—which is based on studies of the genetics of viruses and bacteria, and how these tiny organisms can be made to manufacture human proteins to meet human medical needs.

Essentially, the idea of recombinant DNA technology is to obtain a gene-sized piece of DNA (coding for a single protein) from one organism and introduce (splice) it, functionally intact, into the DNA of another host, such as a bacterium. The host will then manufacture the protein product of the new gene along with its own proteins. The reasoning is that even if the purpose of the inserted gene is unknown, its acceptance and activity in the host—which does not carry that gene—will result in a novel and recognizable protein or protein segment. Using a simple, living organism, such as a bacterium, means that duplicate copies of the successfully transferred gene are made each time the bacterium doubles its DNA before division—so that large quantities of the gene are produced. And the newly programmed bacteria (and their descendants) will, hopefully, churn out the protein ordered by the new gene.

The discovery of how viruses infect bacteria, incorporating their own DNA into a bacterium's, and how bacteria can transfer genes to each other, was made in the 1960s. An important finding in this work, relative to the use of recombinant DNA techniques, was that the ability to "donate" genes to a bacterium was controlled not on the single bacterial chromosome, but on separate, tiny rings of DNA, called plasmids, independently located in the bacterium's cytoplasm.

An important finding of the 1970s was the way bacteria normally fend off foreign intrusions, such as by viruses seeking to integrate their DNA. Bacteria produce scores (and possibly hundreds) of different enzymes, so-called restriction enzymes. Each enzyme guards against a specific short nucleotide sequence—a perceived "nonsense phrase" such as might appear in a piece of foreign DNA. If this antagonistic sequence ever appears in bacterial DNA, the enzyme cuts into it, cutting loose and inactivating the foreign fragment, thus destroying the intruder.

Plasmids and restriction enzymes have become valuable tools for the insertion into bacteria of genes whose cloning is desired. Plasmids can be separated by centrifugation from bacteria. Likewise, restriction enzymes, which do not require living hosts and are functional when removed from the cells, can be isolated. A given plasmid is likely to be cut open in one or several places when dipped into a container of various restriction enzymes, so that the circular DNA will open up, presenting two ends onto which the new gene can be tacked. The new gene to be inserted is given flanking nucleotides that will couple with these end strands. Another enzyme is added to glue the foreign gene into place. The altered, or recombinant, plasmids can readily be re-inserted into the bacterial host by mixing the two together in the presence of calcium ions, causing the bacteria's outer coats to become permeable, and allowing the hybrid plasmids to slip in.

To be of value, a given gene must be able to be produced in the desired quantity; its incorporation into a simple biological system (living or quasi-living) that replicates and divides is a logical method. The bacteria are kept healthy and dividing in nutrient-stoked fermentation vats; and the plasmids' DNA is replicated whenever the bacteria's chromosomal DNA replicates. The plasmids are given laboratory help to assure the new gene's expression (i.e., the production of the new protein). Scientists can also engineer DNA control regions into the bacteria along with the new gene. These sequences, recognized as "start" and "stop" nucleotide phrases by the bacterium, set the boundaries for the make-up of the new protein. The products of the newly expressed gene can be harvested from the bacterial factories (see Figure 13).

There are several ways of obtaining the desired gene. The most laborious process, only practical for tiny proteins, is the laboratory synthesis of genes by painstaking assembly of nucleotide building blocks whose sequence has been determined by analysis of the protein for which it codes. With the aid of a restriction enzyme from one bacterium, plasmids from another bacterium are cut open. The synthesized gene and an appropriate control region are then grafted onto the host bacteria's plasmids. *A successful example of this technique is the production of human growth hormone.*

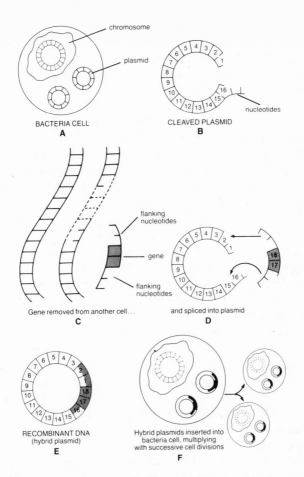

Figure 13. Diagram of gene-splicing, or recombinant DNA, process. A bacteria cell (A), containing a single chromosome and a few free-floating DNA rings called plasmids, is broken open and the plasmids are removed. The plasmids are split open with a special enzyme (a bacterial restriction enzyme) that cleaves a specific nucleotide sequence (B). Using the same restriction enzyme, a DNA segment containing a gene-sized sequence from another organism (such as a human gene) is cleaved at the same nucleotide sequence, thus leaving the gene with flanking nucleotides that will correspond with the open ends of the plasmid (D). Another enzyme is used to seal the new gene and its flanking nucleotides into the plasmid, forming a hybrid plasmid (E). The hybrid plasmids are inserted into other bacteria (F), and will be replicated along with the bacterium's chromosomal DNA, and will multiply with successive divisions of the bacterial cells. Hopefully the new gene will be expressed in the host bacterium, which will churn out the gene's ordered protein product. (*Harvey Offenhartz, Inc.*)

Another technique for obtaining a single gene is to isolate messenger RNA—the executor-intermediary responsible for taking the instructions from the gene and "translating" them into the protein product—from cells or tissues known to be abundant synthesizers of the desired protein. The isolated RNA is then mixed with free nucleotide building blocks and the enzyme called reverse transcriptase. As discussed earlier, this enzyme, found in RNA viruses, allows the viruses to use their own genetic material—RNA only—as the template for new DNA in the host cell. In a reverse of the usual process—DNA being used as a blueprint for the manufacture of RNA—the RNA segment, with the aid of reverse transcriptase, can order the construction of a strand of DNA complementary to itself. The DNA replicates itself into double-stranded DNA, and a potentially functioning gene is formed. The new gene is then inserted into bacteria for processing, via the plasmid techniques. *This is the technique used to synthesize human insulin, first accomplished in 1979.*

The third method of obtaining genes has been called the "shotgun" approach. The entire six-foot thread of DNA from a human cell is snipped into gene-sized fragments by restriction enzymes. Each of the DNA fragments, likely to be an integral gene but of unknown function, is separately inserted into a piece of the DNA of viruses known to infect bacteria; the viral DNA serves as the transfer vehicle, in place of a plasmid. This doctored viral DNA, each piece presumably linked with a gene-sized fragment of human DNA, is then inserted into bacteria—one human-viral hookup per bacterium. Each hybrid bacterium is grown into a colony in a separate dish containing growth medium. The dishes housing each bacterium are then tested one by one, to find the colony making the desired product; the responsible human-viral DNA combination can be isolated, and the successful gene extracted. *This technique, and the screening of thousands of bacteria cultures, were part of the method that led to the identification and isolation of the human gene coding for interferon—a potent antiviral agent to be discussed later.*

In the mid-1970s, as the potential of gene splicing and genetic engineering began to be realized, there was considerable concern and controversy about such laboratory creations—in the scientific community as well as among legislators and the public at large.

Visions of mutant bacteria, possibly equipped with virulent DNA and new genes that conferred drug resistance (and thus protection against destruction), escaping from laboratories and wreaking havoc, resulted in stringent guidelines by the National Institutes of Health for the types of mutations (or recombinants) that could be formed or attempted.

These restrictions have since been relaxed, for a number of reasons. For one, the bacteria used in this work are special, weakened strains, bred to require "laboratory fare"—nutrients not available in the outside world. An animal or human host could not provide the right nourishment; and if these bacteria somehow invaded a human host, say a laboratory worker, the bacteria would die within a few hours. Further, the chances of pieces of the working material—free genes or segments of viral DNA—escaping and finding a conducive home on the chromosomes of an animal or human are infinitesimal.

Currently, only about 15 percent of all work with recombinant DNA falls into the category of presenting possible "biohazards." Researchers conducting such possibly hazardous studies must first submit planned safeguards against the dangers, and have their cautionary measures approved by their own institution and then by the National Institutes of Health or any other organization from which they receive research funding.

Gene-Splicing Potential for Medical Application

A number of substances synthesized by genetically engineered microorganisms are currently being tested for therapeutic potential in patients. The products include interferon; insulin; human growth hormone; an anti-inflammatory hormone called ACTH; a hormone called calcitonin, which is used to treat degenerative bone disease; blood factors for the treatment of hemophilia; an enzyme called urokinase used to dissolve blood clots; the hormone thymosin, which shows promise as a treatment for brain and lung cancer; and a large peptide (protein) called an endorphin, a powerful pain killer. Some fifty other hormones and small proteins, according to the U.S. Congress's Office of Technology Assessment, may be produced by gene-splicing technology within an estimated five to ten years.

The value of such production methods is that they will make potentially important treatment agents available in large quantities and at a low cost—crucial factors for testing and application. Such engineered products, as compared to naturally occurring extracted substances, can also be "ordered" by genes that have been trimmed or enhanced to make a product of greater purity and potency, with minimal side effects.

It is theoretically possible to clone (i.e., isolate and nurture the proliferation of) any of the gene-sized DNA segments in a human cell. It has already become possible, using gene-splicing techniques and bacterial factories, to produce large quantities of many small proteins (such as peptide hormones) that are the direct end products of a particular gene whose coding sequence is short and whose processing requires only a few, uncomplicated enzyme assists.

For more complex proteins, the production of a bona fide or useful duplicate is much more difficult, and years away from accomplishment. These are proteins whose gene-coding sequences may be functionally linked to others; which may contain numerous nonexpressed but vital regulatory DNA segments; whose transcriptions may proceed in separate cascade "runs" and may require many enzyme-processing steps for completion; or whose expression may require the presence of other stimulatory chemical signals.

However, there are numerous research projects underway where streamlined, synthetic genes are being used, via gene splicing into bacterial hosts, to code for relatively complex proteins. Some of these appear to carry instructions for a more pure and potent product—*without* all the native nucleotide baggage. Similarly, manipulated mutations in the natural genetic makeup of microorganisms that are sources of useful drugs have permitted a higher yield of the desired substance by eliminating "extraneous" DNA activity.

For example, chemically induced mutations in a strain of the *E. coli* bacteria used to produce the anti-leukemia enzyme, asparaginase, improved the enzyme yield over 100 times that of the original bacteria strain. The cost of a course of asparaginase therapy was lowered from nearly $15,000 to about $300.

There are a number of proteins whose manufacture in quantity could lead to dramatic progress in cancer therapy. Potential candidates for production in the foreseeable future, by gene-splicing technology and cloning via microorganisms or possibly via cells of higher animals, are the peptide hormones thymopoietin, which stimulates the differentiation of T lymphocytes; and erythropoietin, which stimulates production of red blood cells; and a range of immune-system proteins. These immunoproteins, which will be further discussed in this chapter's section on immunology, include: antigens specific to malignant cells that can be rendered harmless and used as vaccines to prime an individual's response against actual malignant cells; interferons and other lymphokines, active regulatory molecules vital to an energetic immune response; antibodies, including tumor-specific varieties; and enzymes, whose absence or abnormality is known to cause a number of diseases.

The advances in genetic engineering and gene mapping will allow a much more focused investigation of the processing and production of important and complex proteins. These advances offer valuable tools for understanding what is missing (or "turned off"), redundantly repeated, misplaced, or abnormally present in the DNA of persons with hereditary diseases or acquired diseases that can be traced to abnormal DNA coding.

Transcriptions of the order of nucleotide bases in a "responsible" gene linked to a particular disease can be compared to the same DNA segment from normal cells. This has already been done with sickle-cell anemia and a type of anemia in which hemoglobin leaks from red blood cells (a disease known as thalassemia); and matching techniques now allow for prenatal screening for these diseases.

Other adaptions of gene-splicing technology are geared to the introduction of novel and advantageous genes, such as those that might confer disease resistance or drug resistance, from one laboratory animal to another. In one application of this sort, researchers at UCLA spliced DNA segments with repetitive copies of a gene coding for an enzyme whose overabundant presence rendered mice resistant to methotrexate, the anti-leukemia drug, from one line of mice into a different (but immunologically compatible) line of mice whose bone marrow had been destroyed by irradiation, and which had been injected with a mixture of the new genes and donor marrow from yet another immunologically compatible line of mice.

The "take" could be demonstrated by the presence in recipient mice of only donor cells, and the ability to withstand doses of methotrexate that would destroy normal cells. Many of the recipient mice, under this pressure for survival, began rapidly cloning any methotrexate-resistant cells. The research proved that the desired DNA could be incorporated into the cells of other animals; and that some of these transformed cells could be functional in still another animal.

These findings may eventually be of use in helping patients undergoing chemotherapy. The technique would involve removing healthy bone marrow cells from a patient during remission (or from an immunologically compatible donor) and transforming them with engineered genes that will induce resistance to the treatment drug. The transformed cells could be given back to the patient during a course of high-dosage (and normally lethal) chemotherapy that would wipe out all marrow cells with the exception of the resistant cells, which would be normal and preferentially survive.

Among the most exciting medical potentials of gene mapping and genetic engineering is the possibility of transferring normal human genes into human cells, with the aim of establishing a take-over line of competent cells in a person with a genetic structural or metabolic defect of serious consequence.

For example, cells that normally express the desired gene could be taken from a patient with a defect in the gene's expression, e.g., by extracting pancreatic islet cells from a diabetic patient; the faulty but appropriate cells could be spliced and rid of the defective gene, with normal insulin-coding genes grafted in their place. The doctored cells would then be reinjected into the pancreas, hopefully to thrive, secrete insulin, obey the signals of the cell's regulatory genes, and respond appropriately to other chemical stimuli or inhibitors (e.g., the grafted insulin gene should respond to changing blood glucose levels).

This scenario is visionary, and not yet even a technical possibility; but scientists believe that such capabilities are forthcoming. Initial attempts to introduce functional foreign human genes, produced by accepting microorganisms, into human cells were made in 1980, but were not successful. Most researchers believe it will take at least several years and considerable groundwork before normal human genes introduced into patients form colonies of cells that can compensate for defective ones. At present, there is no way to integrate a gene into a specific chromosome, even with its location mapped; nor is there any way to guarantee its expression. Just as important, the gene, were it to be integrated and expressed, would have to be attuned to the cell's—and the body's —regulatory mechanisms.

IMMUNOLOGY AND IMMUNOTHERAPY

The essential objectives of basic research in immunology related to leukemia and other malignancies are: (1) to understand why a patient's immune-response system does not recognize or does not destroy malignant cells; and (2) to find ways to stimulate such activity or compensate for its lack. Clinical trials using immunotherapy, as introduced in chapter 3, focus on two major approaches: (1) injecting the patient with substances that will generate maturation, provoke combative action, or spur greater productivity of white blood cells; and (2) injecting the patient with extracted, synthetic, or "engineered" substances that may override immune-response lacks, compensating the patient with chemicals that protect normal cells, duplicate their products, or aid in the immune attack against abnormal cells.

Sometimes immunotherapy has a dual effect in cancer patients; that is, a substance may stimulate the patient's immune system at the same time it compensates for weak links in the system. Put another way, immunotherapy may either directly *stimulate* components of the immune system or *mimic* products that would accompany an immune attack, thereby stimulating activation responses in white blood cells. The latter approach is the biological equivalent of introducing smoke, so that white blood cells will seek out the fire.

The main areas of activity in immunology and immunotherapy relevant to leukemia treatment today include:

169

1. The use of replacement or booster substances that are biologically active regulators of cells involved in an immune response; these are the so-called "biological response modifiers."
2. Manipulation of leukemic cells to render them more immunogenic (i.e., capable of eliciting an immune response) in a host who has demonstrated unresponsiveness. One technique of promise involves "unmasking" leukemic cells and using them as a kind of vaccination.
3. The use of monoclonal antibodies against leukemic cell structures or products. It is now possible to create, in the laboratory, selective antibodies against a specific target structure—a cell-surface antigen, or virtually any substance of a degree of chemical complexity to qualify as an antigen.
4. The cloning of particularly effective malignant-cell killers from among a remission patient's array of T lymphocytes. Expanded colonies of proven "effector" T cells could then be used to heighten a patient's immunity to his or her own leukemic cells.
5. Isolation and nurtured proliferation of a patient's natural killer cells, for return to the patient.
6. Development of techniques for priming donor bone marrow cells against the recipient's leukemic cells, so that immunized marrow will have an antileukemic effect in the recipient, without inducing graft-versus-host disease.

These last three approaches are in early stages of research and will not be amplified in this chapter.

Biological Response Modifiers

In 1979, the National Cancer Institute launched a special program, with an annual budget of some $20 million, to investigate and develop for possible anti-cancer activity natural substances, including bodily regulatory molecules, that affect the activities of the immune-response system. Predominant among the substances being evaluated are the so-called lymphokines, biologically active regulatory proteins released into the blood upon activation of white blood cells.

Lymphokines have been studied in a concentrated way only in the past fifteen years; and some 100 different compounds have since been identified as belonging to the category. In addition, some forty proteins, called cytokines, have been identified as being produced by cells other than leukocytes, but having an effect on them. Important among the cytokines are the thymic hormones, produced by cells lining the thymus gland, that appear critical to the differentiation of immature T lymphocytes.

Genetic engineering will play a key role in allowing the synthesis of adequate quantities of lymphokines for basic research, because most lymphokines are the large and complex molecules known as glycoproteins, and laboratory synthesis by chemical construction is not feasible. Interferon was the first lymphokine to be produced by genetically engineered microorganisms; hopefully, the production of other lymphokines will follow.

Interferons. The interferons have been studied more extensively and have earned special recognition among the lymphokines. They are a family of regulatory molecules, chiefly glycoproteins as far as is presently known. Interferons are normally made in very small amounts by virtually any cells that have a nucleus, in response to exposure to viruses and probably other foreign particles. They were discovered in 1957, following observations that demonstrated the presence of a factor in cells exposed to one virus that prevented successful assaults by other viruses. The name interferon was chosen to indicate a function that interfered with viral production.

Interferons, of which there are believed to be at least twenty different molecular forms within three main family types, now appear to have at least fifteen other important biological effects. In the 1970s studies indicated that among these effects was inhibition of virus-induced cancer in animals, and possible containment of malignant-cell proliferation in humans.

Since the discoveries that there are many different forms of interferon, made by a variety of cell types, interest in using the substance for cancer treatment centered on the forms made by white blood cells—those forms that might well be important components of an immune response. Until 1981, studies of interferon were hampered by its scarcity and expense. Natural interferon was used; it was extracted from large quantities of white blood cells, and available only from a center in Finland, where the extraction technique was developed.

The early trials of this extracted interferon in cancer patients (done in 1978 to 1981) involved small dosages of doubtful purity —since estimated to have been only about 0.1 percent pure. These trials involved only several hundred cancer patients at about ten medical centers, and most of the patients were in advanced stages of their disease. The trials yielded mixed results, and are now believed to be of limited value as far as indicating potential; but there were some positive results in shrinking tumors and delaying recurrences of disease in some patients with bone cancer, breast cancer, lung cancer, skin tumors, and lymphomas. No cancer patients were cured with the extracted interferon.

Since 1981, several biotechnology and pharmaceutical companies have succeeded in producing pure interferon with a predictable structure by splicing human interferon genes into bacteria or yeast cells for cloning. This advance has not only produced a pure substance, but has greatly increased the supply and dramatically lowered its price.

How does interferon work? Studies of the extracted interferon indicated that its synthesis is a response to stimulants which vary according to the type of responding cell (e.g., B and T cells release interferon only in response to antigens that specifically activate them); but viral stimulation seems a common motivation for many types of cells. Its action as a response to viral presence is better understood: it serves as a messenger molecule to cells with which the producing cell normally interacts. The interferon molecule binds to cell-surface receptors and induces, in recipient cells, the production of enzymes that intercept and destroy viral RNA, inhibit viral DNA transcription, or otherwise interfere with viral protein assembly or release. The interferon protein's strongest ability appears to be the induction of an anti-viral state in cells undergoing RNA and protein synthesis (see Figure 14).

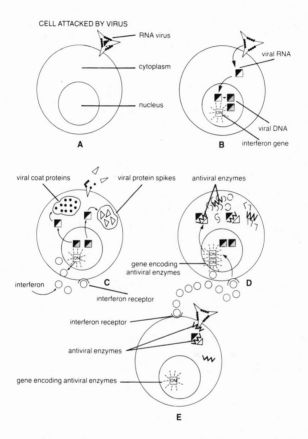

CELL ATTACKED BY VIRUS

Figure 14. Diagram of interferon action. A cell is attacked by a virus (A); the insertion of the virus's genetic material signals the cell to "turn on" its interferon gene (B). The viral DNA succeeds in transcribing RNA that oversees production of viral coat proteins and viral protein spikes (C); but meanwhile interferon is being synthesized, some of which self-stimulates the cell. The interferon stimulus turns on a cellular gene that encodes antiviral enzymes (D), which degrade viral RNA and interfere with viral protein assembly. Molecules of interferon also travel to other cells, bind to interferon receptors, and signal the neighboring cells to produce the antiviral enzymes. *(Harvey Offenhartz, Inc.)*

In the laboratory, cells exposed to interferon express an anti-viral readiness very quickly. But the full anti-viral capability develops gradually over a few hours, and requires that the recipient cell be in the process of protein synthesis—working, not just growing or dividing. Cells that are not working at protein production, but are in phases of growth, DNA replication, or cell division, exhibit an inhibition or even a freeze of these activities.

While specialized activities of mature white blood cells are enhanced by leukocyte interferon (e.g., antibody production is stepped up tremendously), it not only slows or halts growth phases of immature cells, but apparently differentiation phases as well. For this reason the forms of interferon so far studied are totally inappropriate as an eradication treatment for leukemia, since white cells are arrested in their immature, useless stages. It does have potential as a maintenance therapy for leukemia patients, however, because of its ability to stimulate production of antibodies, NK cells, and macrophages.

Interferon is very unstable and its active life is brief; it must be continuously supplied to cells to maintain the anti-viral state, for example. It is all but undetectable a day or two after injection, is quite easily inactivated by various bodily fluids, and does not appear to penetrate the central nervous system readily. This kind of profile applies to many of the body's potent chemicals, such as the complement protein-complex discussed earlier that is kept, biologically, on a short leash to avoid overreactions and excesses which can be dangerous.

Side effects of the interferons, even in the early trials when it was given in small amounts, are fatigue, muscle aches, fever, some hair loss, mild suppression of the marrow's ability to generate blood cells, occasional skin blisters, and toxic effects on the heart in some cases. Researchers caution that the larger dosages that may be necessary for effectiveness against some forms of cancer may also duplicate many of the undesirable side effects of standard anti-cancer drugs.

It seems unlikely that interferon will be a major anti-cancer drug, in terms of eradication potential against established malignancies. "It's disappointing to some, but not surprising to those of us who work in the field, that interferon will not bring miracles as some people once hoped," said Dr. Thomas C. Merigan of Stanford University, one of the pioneers in studying the uses of interferon.*

Several more years will be needed to purify and concentrate the separate forms of interferon; when the various forms are characterized, and if the encoding genes for each can be identified, it is certainly possible that more potent and specific anti-cancer interferons can be produced. The anti-viral properties of the currently available "engineered" interferons can be of great benefit to leukemia and other cancer patients whose immune response has been compromised by radiotherapy or chemotherapy. Interferon has proved itself already to be of prophylactic value against activation of the virus that causes chicken pox, as well as against the herpes simplex virus; this action alone can be lifesaving to many marrow-transplant recipients and other leukemia patients who are lethally threatened by active infections caused by these viruses.

Thymosin. Thymosin, one of the so-called thymic hormones, is naturally produced by epithelial cells lining the thymus gland. Studies indicate that it may be critical to initiating the differentiation process in prothymocytes (immature T lymphocytes), after they arrive in the thymus from the bone marrow. Scientists are working from the laboratory observations indicating that many kinds of cancer cells will respond to external stimuli and differentiate. If the DNA of malignant cells could be signaled to program terminal differentiation (the final phase of maturity for the cell), these cells would no longer be growing and dividing cells, and would be rendered harmless.

Thymosin is a "short" hormone, with only twenty-eight amino acids in its chain, and it can be made by chemical synthesis. It is commercially available, and researchers are studying its potential in animals and in early clinical trials. Proliferation of immature T cells is the immediate problem in about 10 to 15 percent of acute lymphocytic leukemia cases (leukemia identified as T-cell leukemia); and loss of mature T-cell activity against malignant cells, as well as loss of the guidance and regulation by mature T

* "Interferon Makes Inroads Against Some Infections, Including Colds," *The New York Times,* 1 June 1982, pp. C1 and C8.

cells over other cells involved in immune responses, is often the critical deficit in individuals who develop other types of leukemia and other cancers.

T-cell Growth Factor and Macrophage Factors. Activated macrophages and mature T cells release substances (most not yet isolated or characterized) that stimulate growth or differentiation in their own cell line or in leukocytes of other types. One such factor that stimulates the growth of T cells has been isolated from leukocyte cultures of patients with T-cell malignancies. This T-cell growth factor selectively enhances, among mixed normal leukocytes in culture, the growth and perpetuation of normal T cells. The T-cell factor is being purified and characterized, and has not yet been used in clinical trials.

Vitamin A Derivatives. Several synthetic substances that resemble vitamin A are being explored for activity against leukemic cells. For several years, immunologists have noted that vitamin A or synthetics similar in composition appeared to have a nonspecific, enhancing influence on the competence of white blood cells. Under testing for the past few years, some of these analogues of vitamin A have converted, in laboratory dishes, acute myelocytic leukemia cells to a differentiated form that is presumably no longer capable of malignant proliferation. However, not all the derivates (called retinoids or retinoic acids) were effective against the responsive leukemia cells; and many cell samples (collected prior to chemotherapy) from patients with acute leukemia did not respond to any of the analogues.

Laboratory studies are now underway to develop or modify vitamin A analogues that might show consistent differentiation-inducing activity in cell samples from a majority of newly diagnosed acute leukemia patients. Vitamin A itself, and many of the analogues so far tested on animals, have toxic effects in the amounts necessary for bodily influence; these can hopefully be eliminated in modified derivatives.

Lithium Carbonate. In the past several years, various studies of lithium therapy in conjunction with chemotherapy have indicated that lithium stimulates bone marrow stem cells to increase production and undergo differentiation. The effect most prominent in early studies is stimulation of granulocyte formation, which has been advantageous in preventing infections in patients undergoing chemotherapy. Lithium carbonate is a metallic salt that can be toxic in accumulated amounts, so blood levels must be carefully monitored. Its primary use has been to treat manic-depressive mental disorders; elevated granulocyte counts in treated manic-depressives was a chance finding.

The "rescue" potential of lithium to stimulate myeloid stem cells may allow the administration of larger and more curative dosages in chemotherapy. Limited clinical trials are recently underway; and basic research studies continue in search of characterizing lithium's mode and range of action in enhancing the immune response.

Granulopoietin. Scientists at the Bob Hipple Laboratory for Cancer Research of the Wright State University School of Medicine have discovered a natural hormone that regulates the production of granulocytes. This hormone, granulopoietin, was found to increase white blood cell production in laboratory animals. Dr. Martin J. Murphy, Jr., director of the Bob Hipple Laboratory, suggested that granulopoietin might be used to spur production of granulocytes in cancer patients whose normal white blood cell production has been depressed by anti-cancer drugs, leaving them susceptible to deadly infections. The discovery of this hormone might also lead to insights into the mechanisms whereby white blood cells multiply widely, resulting in leukemia.*

Vaccination With Leukemic Cells

In the routine vaccinations of humans against microorganisms that cause serious disease, the aim is prevention: individuals are inoculated with solutions containing killed pathogens or live but relatively harmless varieties of the pathogens. This allows the immune system to establish adequate levels of antibodies and a population of B and T lymphocytes primed to react and multiply should the microorganism ever appear in natural and virulent form.

Vaccination against cancer originated in the late 1960s, when investigators at several institutions tried to stimulate immune re-

* Harold M. Schmeck, Jr., "Key Hormone Is Discovered," *The New York Times*, 21 June 1983.

activity against leukemic cells in patients undergoing maintenance therapy for acute leukemia. The priming bait to induce reactivity was inoculation with another person's leukemic blast cells, irradiated to make them sterile—to confer leukemia-specific immunity, plus a tame form of the tuberculosis bacillus, injected to induce general immune activation.

Irradiated donor leukemic cells showed dubious ability to induce a specific and cell-mediated immune response. Also, current experimental treatments no longer include the use of bacillus extracts, as their effectiveness is uncertain; in fact, some studies indicate that the combination of the bacillus extract with the leukemic cells is statistically less effective than immunotherapy with treated leukemic cells alone. It should be noted that this form of immunotherapy follows remission-induction (complete or partial) with chemotherapy; it is not a primary treatment but a maintenance or adjuvant treatment.

Among the most promising of these vaccination techniques—and more critical in that it involves sustaining remissions for patients with acute myelocytic leukemia, for whom remission maintenance remains a major challenge—is the use of enzyme-modified myeloblastic leukemic cells.

Essentially, the technique involves unmasking the leukemic cells with an enzyme (called neuraminidase) which snips off most of a cell's outermost "branch" molecules—sialic acids—exposing structures more closely bound to the cell's outer membrane. So revealed, the cells stimulate the immune system; and animal studies have shown that recipients primed with these cells could later mount immune responses against *natural* (i.e., not treated with enzymes) leukemic cells.

The cross-reactivity of the inoculations in mice—that is, the immunity conferred on one strain of mice by vaccination with enzyme-treated leukemic cells of another strain—provided the basis for using enzyme-treated allogenic (i.e., coming from others) leukemic myeloblasts as immunity-inducers in patients with acute myelocytic leukemia.

In this technique the myeloblasts of many patients who have been diagnosed as having acute myelocytic leukemia are collected previous to chemotherapy and frozen in liquid nitrogen. Cells are not pooled; one recipient gets a particular donor's cells for at least six months.

On the day of immunotherapy, a supply of cells is thawed, tested for viability, and incubated with purified enzyme (plus calcium, needed for activation of the enzyme). The cells, presumably cleaved of sialic acids, are then washed free of enzyme and used for immunization within an hour. The total immunization dosage in treatments given at Mount Sinai Medical Center in New York is some 100 billion cells, divided among forty-eight injection sites.

Control studies comparing patients treated with maintenance chemotherapy alone to patients treated with chemotherapy plus vaccination immunotherapy, using the enzyme-treated leukemia cells, are less than ten years underway. However, significant differences in remission duration and survivals have already appeared.

In a trial begun in 1973 at Roswell Park Memorial Institute in Buffalo, New York, five patients received maintenance chemotherapy only; and nine received chemotherapy alternating with immunotherapy. All chemotherapy-only patients have died; four patients in the immunotherapy group are still in remission, and five have died.

In trials initiated in 1977 at the Mount Sinai Medical Center in New York City, eighty-six patients with acute myelocytic leukemia in remission are being followed: forty-five of them assigned to receive only maintenance chemotherapy; forty-one of them assigned the protocol of maintenance chemotherapy plus monthly immunotherapy. Results available to date report 24 percent of the patients in the chemotherapy-only group to be still in complete remission, compared to 49 percent of patients in the chemotherapy-plus-immunotherapy group.

In neither of these trials have there been instances of leukemic cell growth or multiplication resulting from the injections. In the Mount Sinai trials, effective sensitization can take up to two years (i.e., priming a patient's immune response, including, it is believed, T cell recognition, in addition to antibody production); and the immunizations are continued for five years.

Patients are injected subcutaneously at forty-eight bodily sites that drain into major lymph node areas in order to get maximum exposure for the immunization cells; such injections take about a half hour and are given monthly. There have been no reported side effects other than transitory lumps at the injection sites.

In the Mount Sinai trials, patients are given skin tests with five common lymphocyte-stimulating antigens about every three months to check skin reactions indicating active immune responsiveness. Their lymphocytees are periodically checked in the laboratory for activity against various antigens; and cell samples are checked for normal proportions among blood cells. Laboratory tests are also conducted periodically to test the activity of their lymphocytes when mixed with samples of their own thawed myeloblasts. The majority of immunotherapy patients show progressively stronger lymphocyte response against their own leukemic cells.

Monoclonal Antibodies

Theoretically, it should be possible to induce antibody formation against any cell mature enough for antigen presentation by exposing that cell to the antibody-producing lymphocytes (B cells) of any other immunocompetent individual with different self-marking or MHC antigens. What if it were possible to then collect those antibodies, which are now programmed to attach themselves to any molecule like the specifically attractive ones on that priming cell? Couldn't the antibodies then be used to stimulate an immune response against the determined target cell-type in any other individual? If the target cell were a cancer cell, couldn't the antibodies be used to help implement an immune response against that type of cancer cell? What if potent poisons were attached to the antibodies, so that they would be even more certain of bringing destruction to the target cell-type? What if radioactive tracers were attached to the antibodies, so that an X-ray of the recipient would show up any pockets of the targeted cancer cells?

While all of these objectives have been theoretically possible, finding ways to make them feasible on demand, under controlled conditions, has only recently been achieved. The centerpiece of this developing technology is monoclonal antibodies.

The groundwork for the development of monoclonal antibodies

was the successful fusion, at the Laboratory of Molecular Biology in Cambridge, England, in 1975, of two types of cells: a mouse lymphocyte that could produce quantities of a single antibody, and a myeloma cell, a malignant counterpart of the lymphocyte. The exciting aspect of this merger was the desirable genetic manifestations in the new fusion cell (named a hybridoma): it secretes the antibody specified by the genes of the normal lymphocyte; and it obeys the genes of the myeloma cell which confer vigorous growth, longevity in laboratory dishes, and a high production rate of the antibody. (Normal lymphocytes do not grow well in culture and have a limited lifespan.)

The next step is to induce the production of antibodies against specific substances that would be antigenic in the mouse. The mouse, injected with the target material, makes antibodies against it, even if specific for only a single chemical phrase of the substance's entire chemical declaration. Although one lymphocyte can make quantities of only a single antibody, other mouse lymphocytes might secrete antibodies against other chemical markers on the same target substance, particularly if the target is a complex one, such as a cell.

Some of the mouse's activated lymphocytes are then extracted and mixed in culture with myeloma cells. Placed in a nutritious growth medium, some of the cells fuse; and some of these, hopefully, will carry the desired genetic mix, providing hale and prolific clones that spill out copious amounts of the antibody specified by the normal lymphocytes. The antibodies can then be harvested (see Figure 15). One obvious criterion in selecting the successful lymphocytes for fusion, with regard to cancer detection or therapy, is that their chosen target on the priming cancer cell be primarily cancer-associated, and only occasionally associated with normal cellular activity; this is now one of the most difficult qualifications to meet.

As a treatment, monoclonal antibodies have been used on an investigational basis only since 1981, in an effort to tag cancer cells with antibodies formed against them. The goal is to induce a follow-through immune response in the patient (i.e., activating T cells, complement, and phagocytes). As with other forms of immunotherapy, monoclonal antibodies are not intended as primary

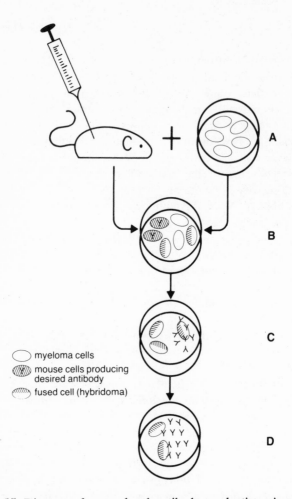

Figure 15. Diagram of monoclonal antibody production. A mouse is injected with a foreign substance, such as human leukemic cells, and will form antibodies against it; some of the mouse's antibody-producing plasma cells are removed (A) and mixed with myeloma cells, malignant counterparts of plasma cells that are of value because of their high production rate of antibodies and their longevity in tissue culture. Some of these cells, in a nutritious growth medium, will fuse (B). The fused cells are separated from the others and examined for those expressing the mouse cell's orders for antibody production (C). These desirably productive cells are isolated and further selected for those that are producing large amounts of the mouse-dictated antibodies (D); these "successful" cells are cloned, and their uniform antibodies harvested for use in immunotherapy. *(Harvey Offenhartz, Inc.)*

treatment against cancer, but, hopefully, they can be a potent partner in stimulating a patient's immune system, perhaps in combination with other forms of treatment.

Early treatment results reported in late 1981 indicated that although the antibodies initially produce a significant drop in malignant cells, the cells eventually lose binding attraction for the antibodies. Often the cells resort to one of the classic evasive strategies of cancer cells: they shed both antibody and antigen from their surfaces, and the antigens reappear when the antibodies are gone. Such "passive" immunizations (the antibodies are given to the patient, not produced by the patient) are only effective for about six months or less, and the patient must receive periodic booster injections.

Partial remissions and encouraging results have been reported among small groups of cancer patients treated with monoclonal antibodies at the Stanford University Medical Center and at the Children's Hospital in Boston. There have been no toxic side effects from the immunizations.

Monoclonal antibodies developed against lymphocytic leukemia cells have been used to treat bone marrow cells in a small number of patients at Children's Hospital. Patients selected were those threatened with relapse, who showed drug resistance, and for whom no compatible donors were available for bone marrow transplants. Three patients are in remission following antibody treatments.

As with standard autologous (self) marrow transplants, these patients had bone marrow removed when they were in remission, to be frozen for future use. However, the marrow was treated before freezing and storage with leukemia-directed monoclonal antibodies. The patients received large dosages of radiation and chemotherapy to kill remaining bone marrow cells, and were "rescued" with infusions of their remission-marrow. Any leukemic cells in the infused marrow would presumably have antibodies attached, and so could stimulate an immune response as the patients' blood cells began to generate. Drug therapy is contra-indicated as it would suppress immune response and bone marrow activity.

During 1983, it is estimated, about a dozen medical centers in the United States will have programs using monoclonal antibodies. It is estimated also that some seventy treatment and research centers and private companies are now undertaking research work with monoclonal antibodies, for diagnosis and/or for treatment of various cancers.

One immediate problem involving target-cell recognition by monoclonal antibodies is the fact the scientists have yet to find antigens that are unique to cancer cells. This is not a problem in *producing* the antibodies, since laboratory animals injected with human malignant cells will naturally form antibodies against such species-foreign cells. The problem will be to screen the produced antibodies for their attraction to cellular products or cell-surface molecules that are only rarely present in normal tissues or cells. Equally important is that the produced antibodies be those that form a strong bond with the antigen; this usually requires that the antibody be able to bind an antigen molecule at several points.

Leukemia cells are believed to often carry "leukemia-associated" antigens, but they are probably "low profile" ones. Experiments in mice using monoclonal antibodies that recognized a thymocyte (immature T cell) antigen showed that the antibodies also recognized injected leukemic cells. The monoclonal antibodies were mixed with complement and injected into mice with leukemia characterized by lymphoblasts that were undoubtedly thymocyte precursors; the treatment induced complement and granulocyte elimination of the leukemic cells.

The problem of target specificity is large. Not only must antigen targets be primarily exclusive to malignant cells, but such antigens must also be common to many types of malignant cells. Studies with monoclonal antibodies developed against human leukemia cells have shown distinctions among leukemic cell types that were previously presumed to be uniform.

The potential exists for developing an arsenal of monoclonal antibodies, categorized according to type and even subtype of target malignant cell. It is not farfetched to envision computer match-ups between malignant cells' surface antigens or surface products, and monoclonal antibodies in the arsenal that are specific for these cells' most exclusive chemical attributes.

When potent, pure, cancer-cell antibodies are isolated, large quantities can be produced, either from cultivating the responsible hybridomas in laboratory dishes, or through genetically engineered microorganisms.

Monoclonal antibody research is being directed also at linking potent anti-cancer antibodies (those that are most exclusive and also form stable antigen bonds) with a powerful cell-killing substance. Research is already underway in animals in which monoclonal antibodies are combined with compounds called chelates, which contain highly radioactive metals. The radiation is of a kind that delivers a heavy dose to target cells, but does not penetrate to adjoining tissues. Other investigators are working on attaching anti-cancer drugs to monoclonal antibodies, hopefully to create a "missile" that will seek out and destroy only malignant cells.

The development of an array of potent and highly selective monoclonal antibodies, each targeted against a particular leukemic cell marker, has the potential for an effective maintenance therapy for patients; such antibodies may be particularly effective when combined with immune-system stimulators, now under development. As a curative therapy, the potential for "naked" monoclonal antibodies is limited; but when ways of linking them to poisonous cargo (drugs, radioactive substances) can be developed, they might indeed become guided missiles that can destroy malignant cells.

VIROLOGY

As discussed earlier, the research work with viruses that cause leukemia and other cancers in animals has led investigators to specific "cancer genes" in humans—normally dormant or minimally functional genes that are switched on by viruses and presumably other carcinogens to transform the cell into a malignant automaton. The proteins ordered by these cancer genes are being analyzed with the objective of developing specific chemical antagonists. Even if these transforming proteins are not exclusive to malignant cells, research indicates that malignant cells produce the proteins in far greater quantities than normal cells. This would be a basis for preferential attraction of chemical antagonists, customized to bind to the transforming proteins, and preferential eradication of malignant cells.

PHARMACOLOGY AND CELL KINETICS

Drugs are medically defined as any chemical compounds or noninfectious biological substances used for their functional effects —in diagnosing, treating, or preventing disease or other abnormal, painful, or debilitating conditions. Anti-cancer drugs range from cell poisons and cell "wedges" that block growth or division, to the "biological response modifiers," that might, in force, stimulate the immune system to destroy malignant cells; or, conversely, encourage malignant cells to differentiate or mature and thereby convert to normal.

The trend in drug research today aimed at cancer treatment is to create products that follow the leader—the activated and fully competent immune-response system. As noted in earlier sections of this chapter, the emphasis in this new generation of drugs is to stimulate the immune-response system or to supply chemicals that will overcompensate the patient for lacks in immune-system components or other chemicals that feed into the immune system. Few of these new classes of drugs are yet in clinical trials, except for some of the "biological response modifiers" and a limited range of monoclonal antibodies. Genetic engineering will play a crucial role in obtaining adequate supplies of pure immunoproteins—an inclusive term for all the natural defensive or regulatory proteins that bear on immune response.

In the same way, however, that antibiotics not only aid an individual stricken with a severe bacterial infection, but may be lifesaving, the class of anti-cancer drugs that paralyze or kill malignant cells will continue to be necessary for individuals with a large burden of malignant cells, at least for the foreseeable future. The emphasis in research on this destructive class of drugs is to discover or design drugs that closely fit the profile, activities, or needs of malignant cells, as distinct from normal cells. New or modified drugs of this category are undergoing clinical tests; a number of them are drugs developed or clinically tested in other countries. Particularly encouraging are several new drugs that have shown activity against acute myelocytic leukemia.

No attempt will be made here to list all the drugs undergoing various phases of clinical testing against leukemia in this country or abroad, but a few drugs that seem to show promise are described below:

- Small clinical trials began in 1980 with a drug known as aclacinomycin, an analogue of the anthracycline antibiotic, Adriamycin. Although Adriamycin is effective for induction chemotherapy against both acute lymphocytic and acute myelocytic leukemia, dosages must be limited primarily because of the drug's potential for causing heart damage. In clinical trials in Japan, however, aclacinomycin caused neither heart damage nor hair loss.

- An alkaloid derived from a Chinese evergreen has been recommended for its results against acute myelocytic leukemia by Chinese oncologists. (The only alkaloid, derived from the periwinkle plant, currently in use against leukemia in the United States is vincristine.) Quantities of the drug, known as harringtonin, are now being used in small clinical trials in this country. Preliminary evaluations show the drug to be of limited value, but tests have just started.

- A new drug known as m-AMSA has shown strong activity against acute myelocytic leukemia in patients who had received other treatments and were in relapse. The drug is now undergoing clinical trials as an induction drug for patients newly diagnosed with acute myelocytic leukemia—with impressive results.

There are currently in use in the United States some 120 drugs with proven activity against cancer. Chemical compounds that are recommended for testing are collected from around the world by the National Cancer Institute's chemotherapy research office in Brussels, Belgium, which has acquired over 19,000 chemical compounds and biological substances. Clinical tests, in various phases, are underway on about fifteen drugs each year in the United States;

while some forty drugs, under NCI auspices, are undergoing clinical trials in Europe.

Methods of speeding up evaluations of any drug's probable effectiveness are being refined. The traditional system has been to use immune-suppressed mice, inject them with human malignant cells, then administer the trial drug and check the mice for malignant growth or control; this process takes one to two months.

A method that has proven as equally predictive as the traditional technique involves implanting human malignant cells in a capsule under the kidney in the mouse, a site found to be a sanctuary from immune-system destruction. Growth or shrinkage of the resultant tumor—after a drug is injected—is easily measured, and results of a drug's effectiveness can be obtained within ten days. The NCI predicts that the new method will double the number of compounds (i.e., increase to about thirty) that it can screen each year.

As mentioned in chapter 3, a technique has been developed also to culture human malignant stem cells, and evaluate such cells' abilities to form colonies (self-duplicates and progeny cells), both before and after exposure to a trial drug. Although this method is highly accurate (96 percent) for predicting resistance to drugs (i.e., by observing that colonies continue to form after drug exposure), it is only 62 percent accurate in predicting drug effectiveness in the patient following successful colony-inhibition by the drug in laboratory dishes.

A critical factor in most effective chemotherapy is the synchronization of drug administration with cell-phase readings that indicate when most of a patient's leukemic cells are most vulnerable to destructive drugs, which is when they are preparing for division or in the process of division (see "Checking Chemotherapy Effectiveness," in chapter 3). Researchers are also studying drug potency and effectiveness as influenced by possible modifiers such as ultrasound, in which vibrationally altered cancer cells may become more permeable to drugs; the application of heat; and time of day for optimal drug effectiveness. Little information is available on results of the ultrasound experiments, but heat and biorhythm studies are outlined below.

Hyperthermia

About a dozen medical centers are conducting animal experiments or clinical trials limited to cancer patients with advanced disease, to test the possible enhancement of drug-induced cell kill by hyperthermia (high temperature) treatments. The rationale is that cancer cells have a reduced ability to dissipate heat, and seem in general to have a slightly higher metabolism, and are thus already a little warmer than normal cells. It is thought that by raising body temperature to 107 degrees Fahrenheit, or raising the temperature of local tumors to over 120 degrees, cancer cells would be "cooked" and destroyed, while normal tissues would be spared. Combined with chemotherapy, hyperthermia appears to have a synergistic effect, disrupting the outer membranes of malignant cells and allowing drug penetration, which can make even drug-resistant cells susceptible.

One of the largest studies of hyperthermia on localized tumors has been underway since 1977 at the UCLA Comprehensive Cancer Center, where an instrument called the Magnetrode was developed. The device is a metal ring that can encircle any portion of the body, delivering and inducing electrical currents that generate heat. The treatment, delivered to deep tumors in every part of the body except the brain, and combined with chemotherapy or radiation if the patient's condition permits, has produced tumor regressions and a number of partial remissions, and reduced pain.

Other methods of hyperthermia (combined with chemotherapy) used for systemic cancers involve heating the entire body, or just the blood, up to 108 degrees, the top limit before healthy cells begin to break down. These techniques include dressing the patient in a plastic "space suit" through which 107-degree water flows; bathing the patient in hot wax; and shunting the patient's blood through a heater.

Chemotherapy and Circadian Rhythms

Metabolic and other physiological activities of the body have a rhythmic biological synchronicity that is known as circadian ("about the day") rhythm. A person's vital signs, hematocrit, blood glucose level, and even internal eye pressure vary at different times of the day. There is also variation of activity at any given time of day among individuals, for "night owls" as compared to "early birds," for example. Researchers are now investigating the link between timing of drug administrations and the effectiveness of drug action.

In studies with mice, researchers inoculated twelve different groups with over four million leukemic cells per mouse, a dose that would be lethal in six days, without treatment. Then each group was given three anti-leukemic drugs sequentially, each group receiving its drugs at a different time. The mice who received their last dosage at 5:00 A.M. had a 52 percent cure rate; while groups who had the same drug given at 8:00 or 11:00 A.M., or 2:00 or 8:00 P.M., had a cure rate of only 16 percent. Tests in mice have also shown varying rates of toxicity from drugs, depending on the time of day they are administered.

Some clinical trials are now underway to test possible optimal times of day for chemotherapy for cancer patients. Although preliminary results at the University of Minnesota with the administration-timing of Adriamycin (an anti-leukemia drug also used for some other kinds of cancer) indicate that the drug is indeed metabolized differently when given to patients at 6:00 A.M. as compared to 6:00 P.M., no definitive guidelines for effectiveness according to timing can yet be drawn.

To review, the main approaches in developing anti-cancer drugs today are: (1) designing drugs that are selectively attracted to or preferred by malignant cells—and that will inactivate or kill them; (2) using genetically engineered microorganisms to produce in quantity the missile-like monoclonal antibodies that have been programmed to bind to structures exclusive or highly specific to malignant cells, flagging the cells for the immune system, or killing the cells outright, when lethal payloads are attached to the antibodies; (3) discovering and categorizing molecules associated with inducing or maintaining malignant transformation of cells— i.e., "cancer genes" and their protein products—and developing drugs that inactivate or inhibit these structures, or kill cells that contain them; (4) providing to cancer patients large quantities of

natural regulatory or defensive substances made by the body—
i.e., the growing family of "biological response modifiers"; and
(5) increasing the arsenal of support drugs, those that counter
infection, protect normal cells, or stimulate blood-cell production.

The dual objective of the new generation of anti-leukemia drugs
is to discover or design lethal keys that fit the biochemical locks
exclusive to leukemic cells; and to provide patients with drugs that
biochemically exhort white blood cells to vigilance or action, and
caution other cells to protect their integrity.

The philosophy of the first objective was simply put by Dr.
Christian de Duve, a Nobel Prize-winning biologist at New York
City's Rockefeller University: "Look at it this way; if you want
to get rid of your rich uncle, and he drinks gibsons while everyone
else takes martinis with a twist, you poison the onions, not the
gin."*

One of the newest routes to this objective, not yet discussed in
this chapter, is taking advantage of computer science.

Designing Drugs with Computers

In universities and pharmaceutical companies, chemists and
biophysicists are now working together to create images of molecules on computer screens, keying-in information on a molecule's
structure, volume, and electrical charges. The aim is to visually
and then actually tailor drug molecules to molecules of a disease-
causing substance. This sophisticated objective takes into account
not only the respective molecules' structural and chemical attraction, but aspects of "fit" that scientists in the past few years have
found to be crucial to chemical reactivity and bonding: three-
dimensional correspondence and compatible electrical fields (i.e.,
"sharing" of electrons).

Scientists at the Washington University School of Medicine in
St. Louis are attempting to design steroidlike molecules that will
specifically seek out enzymes that are strongly suspected of stimulating malignant-cell growth—e.g., the products of the so-called

* "Drugs Against Cancer," *Newsweek*, 1 April 1975, pp. 52–53.

"cancer genes." The makeup of the synthetic steroid will be such that when it locks into the enzyme, the ensuing chemical reaction will destroy both the enzyme and the steroid. These studies are in early stages, with the synthetic steroids being tested in bacteria and rats.

Scientists at Rensselaer Polytechnic Institute in Troy, New York, are using computers to analyze anti-cancer drugs and possible synthetics that will bind to DNA—specifically, drugs that wedge themselves between nucleotides, preventing the DNA from transmitting its message. Some of their designed molecules are now being tested by the NCI for anti-cancer effectiveness and safety.

Cancer-Preventive Drugs

The second objective of the pharmacological attack against leukemia and other cancers—"beefing up" the immune-response system—has been covered in this chapter. One offshoot of this "accentuate the positive" approach that has not yet been discussed is protection of cell integrity against malignant transformation.

The NCI has categorized as "chemopreventive agents" certain new drugs or natural substances that have shown promise in cell cultures or in animals in preventing, interrupting, or inhibiting malignant changes or potential in cells. The synthetic analogues of vitamin A, which have shown potent activity against cancer cells in culture—actually inducing them to mature—were discussed earlier in this chapter in the section on immunology.

Natural antioxidants (which prevent the loss of electrons from molecules' electrical fields), such as vitamin C and vitamin E, may play a role in maintaining the integrity and reactivity of surface molecules in cells. Used prophylactically, such substances could prevent or inhibit malignant changes—and have been found to do so in cell cultures. A synthetic antioxidant, known as butylated hydroxyanisole (BHA) has been found in the laboratory to inhibit cancer induced by almost every category of chemical carcinogen. BHA's mode of action is to stimulate two major enzymes that can break up and detoxify carcinogens.

The use of vitamins or synthetic analogues cannot exert much influence when the body's burden of malignant cells is large. However, as an adjuvant or follow-up treatment for patients in complete or partial remission, such drugs could prove significantly helpful in preventing cancer recurrence.

OTHER CLINICAL RESEARCH STUDIES AND APPLICATIONS

Several areas of research that don't fit under the broad categories of anti-cancer drugs, immunotherapy, and the innovations in genetics, are nonetheless important as they affect the individual patient's prognosis and quality of life. Several of these topics are covered below.

Tailoring Chemotherapy and Patient Prognosis

As introduced in chapter 3, patient "profiles" are very important in assigning patients to treatment schedules, and in establishing for the patient, his or her family, and the attending physicians, realistic expectations of leukemia treatment within today's capabilities. A growing number of leukemia treatment centers are applying to each patient a checklist of significant "prognosis factors" that allows treatment decisions which will avoid dangerously overtreating a patient who is likely to respond well to standard regimens, or dangerously undertreating patients who need aggressive or experimental programs if remission is to be attained and sustained. A number of prognostic indicators, involving laboratory studies and patient characteristics, have been drawn up in recent years at several leading leukemia centers. Following is a compiled list of the factors and differentials that are considered important in deciding the course of treatment, and in evaluating a patient's chances of winning the fight against leukemia.

Children with Acute Lymphocytic Leukemia
  1. Pretreatment factors indicating favorable response
     to standard chemotherapy, and likelihood of sus-

tained remission: age between three and seven; white blood cell count below 10,000 per milliliter of sample; normal levels of antibodies in the blood; leukemic cells small and with scanty cytoplasm.

2. Pretreatment factors indicating a less favorable response to standard chemotherapy, and likelihood of relapse: age under three or over seven; white blood cell count over 20,000; low levels of antibodies in the blood; large leukemic cells, with ample cytoplasm; lymph node enlargement; enlarged spleen and liver; 20 percent or more of leukemic bone marrow cells have surface markers characteristic of precursors of T cells (i.e., thymus-derived lymphocytes).

3. Differentials based on response to induction chemotherapy point to rapidity of remission induction—by day fourteen of chemotherapy—as a favorable indicator of a lengthy remission or possible cure.

Adults with Acute Myelocytic Leukemia

1. Pretreatment factors associated with a favorable response to chemotherapy: age under sixty; low blood levels of the enzyme known as lactic dehydrogenase; a favorable ratio of mature myeloid cells (i.e., all white cells other than lymphocytes) to blast cells or myeloid precursor cells; absence of infection at the time of evaluation; stimulated leukemic stem cells in culture do not multiply or form only small aggregates of less than twenty cells; leukemic stem cells in culture are inhibited, after introduction of anti-leukemia drugs, from forming colonies.

2. Pretreatment factors associated with a poor response to chemotherapy and the need for aggressive or experimental treatments: age over sixty; high blood levels of lactic dehydrogenase; a poor ratio of mature myeloid cells to blast cells or myeloid precursor cells; presence of infection at the time of evaluation;

stimulated leukemic stem cells in culture form aggregates of more than twenty cells; leukemic stem cells in culture, after introduction of anti-leukemia drugs, continue to form colonies.

Chemotherapy and Parenthood

A report issued in 1980 by the National Cancer Institute, based on a survey over a ten-year period of 448 cancer patients treated with chemotherapy at the NCI's clinical center, had encouraging news for patients who are hopeful of becoming parents. Even high-dose chemotherapy with multiple drugs did not produce harmful effects in infants conceived by patients, both male and female, subsequent to treatment.

Of the female patients followed, it appears that chemotherapy after the first three months of pregnancy does not jeopardize their infants. Women in this group, as well as those who conceived following cessation of chemotherapy, numbered twenty-eight; none of the babies were premature and all had normal birth weights. The study concludes that in most cases the children born to these twenty-eight mothers were normal.

Protection Against Viral Infections

Interferon and several new drugs active against infections by herpes simplex viruses may spare the lives of thousands of leukemia and cancer patients each year—patients in the precarious phases of their treatment when anti-cancer drugs suppress the immune-response system and runaway infections can cause severe complications and even death. Interferon is undergoing patient trials evaluating its benefit in combating chicken pox in patients undergoing chemotherapy; and the herpes drugs are used to curtail active infections by the virus types that ordinarily cause fever blisters or venereal sores but that can ravage vital organs in immune-suppressed patients.

Infection with chicken pox (caused by a herpes virus called

varicella-zoster) in children undergoing chemotherapy (including remission maintenance therapy) can cause life-threatening illnesses such as pneumonia, encephalitis (inflammation of the brain), and hepatitis. A study reported early in 1982 compared the consequences of chicken pox infections in two groups of children undergoing treatment for cancer—those who received interferon injections and those who did not. Although several patients in both groups died of consequences of the viral infection, of those who survived, none who received interferon developed life-threatening complications, and of those who were not treated with interferon, half developed serious complications. Antibodies against the varicella-zoster virus, isolated from persons recently recovered from chicken pox, are also being used to provide temporary protection.

Although most people harbor latent herpes viruses of the type that causes fever blisters (an estimated 90 percent of Americans), and a growing number—estimated at a half a million Americans each year—have contracted genital herpes (known medically as herpes simplex type 2), the phase of infection described as flare-ups, where the virus is actively multiplying and manufacturing its viral proteins, is the life-threatening phase for immune-suppressed patients. As noted in chapter 3, active herpes infections in immune-suppressed patients can seriously affect the respiratory system, brain, and liver.

One of the new herpes drugs is an antimetabolite called Acyclovir; it offers cells that are actively infected with viruses fake viral nucleotides, so that the viral DNA built with these nucleotides can't function and the virus can't reproduce. A study done at Johns Hopkins Oncology Center in Baltimore evaluated the effectiveness of Acyclovir in patients awaiting bone marrow transplants —all known to harbor latent herpes simplex viruses. Researchers found that none of the patients who received Acyclovir (three days before and ten days following the transplant) developed herpes blisters, the tell-tale sign of active infection; while seven of the ten patients who did not receive the drug developed blisters.

Approved by the FDA in late 1982 was another anti-herpes drug called Zovirax, which is activated only when it comes in contact with an enzyme specific to cells infected with the virus; when activated the drug kills the infected cells, but does not damage other cells. Clinical tests at the University of North Carolina showed cancer patients treated with Zovirax had an 80 to 90 percent reduction in the duration of flare-up symptoms.

Also announced in late 1982, but not yet in human trials, is a vaccine against herpes simplex, developed at the University of Chicago. It does not combat active herpes infections, but is intended to protect against them; the vaccine is made of genetically engineered, harmless herpes simplex viruses that will antagonize and prime the immune system but cannot produce disease.

Interferon is also being tested against herpes infections in immune-suppressed patients.

GLOSSARY

The definitions in this glossary are not strict translations from the medical dictionary, but present the words used in the book in terms more readily understandable by those without medical or biological-science backgrounds.

The particular generic or trade-name drugs described or referred to in the book will not be individually defined, although categories of drugs will be. To look up a specific drug, refer to the listing in chapter 3 or check the index.

ACUTE GRANULOCYTIC LEUKEMIA   See *Acute myelocytic leukemia.*

ACUTE LEUKEMIA   Includes all forms of leukemia (proliferations of abnormal and nonfunctional white blood cells) that are characterized by rapid onset—ranging from a few weeks to several months—and rapid progression, resulting in death in three to five months, if not treated.

ACUTE LYMPHOCYTIC LEUKEMIA   The type of leukemia most prevalent in children. This disease involves the aberrant proliferation of immature and nonfunctional lymphocytes. These abnormal cells supersede all or most normal blood components in the bone marrow, and often predominate in the blood as well, before treatment. The peak incidence of acute lymphocytic leukemia occurs in children between two and four years of age.

ACUTE MYELOCYTIC LEUKEMIA (also known as myelogenous or granulocytic leukemia)   The type of leukemia that originates in the blood stem cells called myeloid, the parent cells of all blood cells other than lymphocytes. The disease involves an aberrant proliferation of grossly immature or somewhat differentiated myeloid cells (often called myeloblasts, which take over the bone marrow and often predominate in the blood as well, before treatment. The highest incidence of acute myelocytic leukemia is in those forty-five and older; it can occur in younger adults and children.

ALKALOIDS A group of nitrogen-containing organic substances found in plants. Many are pharmacologically active, such as the alkaloid obtained from the periwinkle plant, used to arrest cell division in leukemia treatment; as well as nicotine, caffeine, and cocaine.

ALKYLATING AGENTS A category of drugs used to treat malignant diseases; highly reactive and fast-acting, these compounds (called "cell poisons") destroy leukemic cells by locking onto the chemicals in DNA, paralyzing the cell's functioning. They preferentially attack cells that are dividing.

ALLOGENIC TRANSPLANT See *Bone marrow transplant.*

AMINO ACIDS A class of organic compounds that are the building blocks of proteins; there are over thirty in all and twenty common ones, several of them essential in human nutrition. These acids are joined together in sequences that determine the nature of each protein. Asparagine was the first naturally occuring amino acid to be discovered (1806).

ANALOGUE A chemical compound with a structure similar to that of another, but differing with respect to a certain component. In medical science, analogues are often inactive compounds intended to defraud cancer cells, such as the antimetabolites; or they are compounds that share the essential activity of another, but lack undesirable components (such as those that may have toxic effects).

ANEMIA An abnormally low number of red blood cells or an abnormally low amount of appropriately transported hemoglobin; anemias range from temporary situations, such as blood loss or dietary deficiencies, to genetically controlled abnormalities in red cell or hemoglobin production or function.

ANTIBIOTICS Substances produced, often through fermentation, by fungi, bacteria, and other microorganisms that suppress the growth of other species of microorganisms. Some can be synthesized in the laboratory, but most are too complex, and the series of biological steps in their production has yet to be elucidated. A special class of antibiotics, called the anthracycline antibiotics, have proven effective against leukemia and other types of malignancy.

ANTIBODY A protein made and released by lymphocytes of the type known as B cells or plasma cells. An antibody is formed in response to the presence in the body of substances the lymphocytes perceive as "non-self" and therefore unwanted—substances that are either foreign to the body's normal supplies or architecture (particularly complex organic structures such as proteins or whole cells), or are abnormally constructed self-parts, such as malignant or defective cells. A structure that attracts an antibody is called an antigen. A particular antibody binds to a specific antigen, chemically neutralizing it and flagging it for destruction by other components of the immune response. Also termed immunoglobulins, antibodies have a characteristic "Y" shape under the microscope; a "constant" portion that identifies them (as one of the five known classes of antibodies: Ig (immunoglobulin) A, IgM, IgG, IgD, and IgE); and a "variable" portion that determines their specific antigen-binding capability. It is estimated that humans can make about a million different antibodies, which are found usually in the blood and in bodily secretions such as saliva and tears. A normal level of blood antibodies is about fifteen milligrams per milliliter of blood.

ANTIGEN A large molecule, usually a protein or a protein-carbohydrate, existing in a free or bound state (as when it's part of the surface structure of a cell). When perceived as a foreign structure by an individual's immune-response system, an antigen will stimulate the production of an antibody that will bind specifically with itself. See also *Histocompatibility antigens*.

ANTIMETABOLITE In the treatment of malignant diseases, a drug that structurally resembles a component or nutrient needed by the cell for energy or growth. A fraudulent building chemical, it is taken in by the cell and sabotages the production of normal cell products and prevents cell activity. Although this class of drugs does not specifically inhibit malignant cells (to the exclusion of normal cells), cells that are in growth stages, as malignant cells often are, are preferentially suppressed.

APLASTIC ANEMIA   A type of red blood cell deficiency that is traced to abnormalities in the blood-generating cells (i.e., stem cells) of the bone marrow. There are usually dangerously low levels of other blood components as well. The condition is difficult to treat adequately.

ASPARAGINASE   An enzyme synthesized by cells that allows the production of a nutrient (the amino acid asparagine) essential to protein building. A fraudulent, similar enzyme is used in leukemia treatment: it exploits the inability of many leukemic cells to produce asparagine by supplying them with a fake enabling enzyme, and these cells are selectively inactivated.

AUTOIMMUNITY   Immune responses directed against one's own tissues. Representing hereditary or acquired defects in the genes governing the immune-response system, or hypersensitive overreaction to stimuli perceived as resembling a once-confronted invader, autoimmune conditions include allergies, myasthenia gravis, lupus, rheumatoid arthritis, and several neurological diseases, probably including multiple sclerosis.

AUTOLOGOUS TRANSPLANT   See *Bone marow transplant.*

B CELL   A type of lymphocyte that spends its formative period in the bone marrow, is released into the blood, and matures into a plasma cell capable of producing antibodies.

BACILLUS   A rod-shaped bacterium.

BCG   A "tame" form of the tuberculosis bacillus (named Bacillus of Calmette and Guerin after its discoverers), sometimes used to stimulate the immune system in leukemia patients following the attainment of remission.

BETA RAYS   Electrically charged, penetrating waves released by radioactive elements such as radium, cobalt, and iridium, or produced from other chemicals that have been manipulated by technological "chiseling" to release the charged waves.

BIOLOGICAL RESPONSE MODIFIERS   Natural or synthetic substances, many of them normal bodily regulators of cellular response, that can be used in patients to change—through stimulation, suppression, "circuit breaking," or biological "shortcut"—a level of cellular activity that is under or above normal.

BIOPSY   The removal of a sample of bodily tissue, and its examination, usually under the microscope, for purposes of diagnosis.

BLAST CELLS   A term usually only applied to stem cells or other undifferentiated cells that are uncontrollably reproducing themselves.

BLOOD The fluid that is pumped by the heart and circulates throughout the body via the arteries, veins, and capillaries. It contains more than 100 components and supplies cells with the oxygen and nutrients they must have to function; and carries away carbon dioxide and other wastes. The fluid portion of blood is plasma, and the cellular components are red cells (erythrocytes), white cells (known collectively as leukocytes), and platelets.

BLOOD-COMPONENT TRANSFUSION A supply of blood elements that are separated from most others in the blood and given to patients who are deficient in, or depleted of, those particular elements. New procedures now allow granulocytes, as well as red cells and platelets, to be separated from a donor's blood (in a continuous-flow procedure) for infusion into the recipient, while the bulk of the blood is returned to the donor.

BONE MARROW The spongy meshwork of connective tissue and cellular components that fills the cavities of bones; marrow consists primarily of fat cells and the precursors (stem cells) of the various blood cells.

BONE MARROW TRANSPLANT The infusion of donor marrow cells, usually done like an ordinary blood transfusion, into patients with severe deficiencies or malignancies in marrow stem cells. As a treatment for leukemia, the patient's own marrow is first destroyed with drugs and radiation, in an effort to eradicate all leukemic cells. It is called an *allogenic* transplant if the marrow is donated by another individual (other than an identical twin, who is a *syngenic* donor); it is called an *autologous* transplant when the marrow used is the patient's own, collected and frozen for storage when the patient was in remission.

CANCER Generally defined as any disease characterized by the uncontrolled growth, and spread of, abnormal, nonfunctional cells. There are believed to be about 100 diseases that fall under the umbrella category of cancer.

CANDIDIASIS An infection caused by *candida*, a genus of yeastlike fungus; it is one of the more common but serious infections to which patients undergoing chemotherapy are prone, due to consequent immune suppression.

CARCINOGEN   Any substance proven capable of causing DNA mutations, and thus potentially or actually capable of inducing or contributing to cancer causation.

CATALYST   A substance, which in biological systems is often an enzyme, that facilitates a biochemical reaction without itself being changed.

CELL   The basic living unit that makes up organized tissue, both plant and animal; consists of a circumscribed, organic body containing a nucleus (with some exceptions), cytoplasm, an outer defining membrane, and various internal structures and separating membranes.

CELL CYCLE   In a growing cell, the phases of rest, energy and nutrient build-up, DNA synthesis, and production of RNA and proteins that occur between the formation of the cell by the division of its mother cell, and the division of the cell itself to form two daughter cells.

CELL CULTURE   See *Tissue culture.*

CELL KINETICS   The dynamics and motions of the cell. The term is used particularly to describe the rate of specific changes in the amount of a given cellular factor in a given time; or the rate of change for a given cellular activity, such as when a lymphocyte goes from a quiescent state to an activated state.

CELL DIVISION   See *Mitosis.*

CELL HYBRIDIZATION   See *Hybrids.*

CENTRAL NERVOUS SYSTEM (CNS)   The brain, brain stem, and spinal cord.

CHEMOTHERAPY   Literally meaning treatment with drugs; general usage indicates drug treatment of malignant diseases.

CHROMOSOMES   The threadlike, hereditary components of a cell that organize themselves in the nucleus prior to cell division, and are composed of gene units made up of DNA. In every normal person each cell—except sperm and egg cells—has forty-six chromosomes, appearing as twenty-two equal pairs plus two sex chromosomes.

CHRONIC LEUKEMIA   One of the two major leukemia classifications, in which the accumulation of abnormal and nonfunctional white blood cells progresses less virulently and rapidly than in acute leukemia, the other major classification.

CHRONIC LYMPHOCYTIC LEUKEMIA   The type of chronic

leukemia in which the predominant abnormal cell accumulation is of the lymphocyte branch, or the parent cells of the lymphocyte branch.

CHRONIC MYELOCYTIC (MYELOGENOUS, GRANULO-CYTIC) LEUKEMIA The type of chronic leukemia in which the predominant abnormal cell accumulation is of granulocytes or of the parent cells of granulocytes—called myeloblastic or myeloid cells; the disease is characterized by the presence of a chromosomal abnormality called the "Philadelphia chromosome."

CIRCADIAN RHYTHM The observed phenomenon that bodily metabolism and many other biological processes vary in a synchronized manner at different times of day; researchers are investigating whether the effectiveness of chemotherapy may also vary depending on cellular receptivity or resistance at different times of day.

CLONE An exact copy of the original organism; in biological systems, a clone is a group of genetically identical cells perpetuated through division and descended from a common progenitor cell.

COLONIES In cell biology, colonies are comparatively large (as distinguished from clusters) accumulations of cells distinguished by a common progenitor or a common purpose. Colonies often arise from need, as in the case of cellular trauma or depletion; or through lack of cell regulation, as in colonies of malignant cells.

COMPLEMENT An interdependent group of eleven enzymatic blood proteins that are attracted by and interact with antigen-antibody complexes; complement proteins act synergistically with white blood cells in an immune response, helping to activate, implement, and complete the dissolution of foreign or abnormal substances or cells.

CRYPTOCOCCOSIS A genus of yeastlike fungus that can infect various parts of the body, but has a predilection for the central nervous system, causing meningitis; a serious threat to patients who are immune suppressed due to chemotherapy, the infection can be treated with a fungus-specific antibiotic.

CULTURE With reference to medical or biological science, a culture is the propagation in the laboratory of microorganisms or of living tissue cells in special substances conducive to their growth.

CYCLE-ACTIVE CELL Any cell that is in some phase of growth and differentiation, aimed at maturity and division. For an average human cell, the cycle period from "birth" to division is about forty-three hours.

CYTOFLUOROMETRY A technique for sorting cells and registering their individual dynamic states. This allows a measurement of the cycle phases in cells of a patient's blood sample, and a determination as to when the patient's bodily leukemic cells are in a phase most vulnerable to drugs. The technique can be used also post-treatment to determine whether chemotherapy has been effective in destroying leukemic cells, again by examining cells in a blood sample.

CYTOKINES Substances secreted by cells that influence the activity of other cells; an umbrella term for substances other than the well-known cell regulators such as hormones, or the separately categorized regulators such as lymphokines.

CYTOLOGY The study of cells.

CYTOMEGALOVIRUS A group of highly host-specific RNA viruses that infect rodents, monkeys, and humans, and cause infected cells to become large, with the nucleus containing much more DNA than that of normal cells; it is a difficult virus to control, and can cause life-threatening infection in patients who are immune suppressed due to chemotherapy.

CYTOPLASM The "factory" of the cell, the organic mass between the outer membrane of the nucleus and the cell's defining surface membrane; chemical stores are maintained in the cytoplasm, as well as transport systems and processing centers. Chemical balances in the cytoplasm may also affect functioning in the cell's nucleus and outer membrane.

DIFFERENTIATION In relation to cell biology, differentiation is the process of acquiring the capabilities to perform the specialized tasks characteristic of a mature and fully functional cell of a given type.

DOMINANT In biological systems, a dominant element is the one, of at least two that are in forced competition for a single role, which prevails because it is stronger in the particular situation; for example, one hand, eye, or side of the brain is used over the other for particular tasks. In sets of genes, the dominant gene from one parent will be manifest to the exclusion of that from the other parent.

DNA Deoxyribonucleic acid, the genetic material that is the body's "master blueprint" of heredity. DNA encodes, through expressed genes, the moment-to-moment activities in every cell that help maintain it in a viable state. It is usually found, in higher organisms, as a double-helix of chemical subunits (predetermined but alterable, as through mutation) making up the genes, located on chromosomes and within the cell nucleus. DNA, through its sequences of chemical subunits, tells every cell what it can do and what its daughter cells can become.

DNA TUMOR VIRUS A virus that can cause malignancies, including leukemia, in various species of animals; made up of a packet of DNA wrapped in a protein coat, the virus tries to insert its own DNA into the nucleus and DNA of cells in host organisms that it invades.

ENZYMES Catalytic molecules, usually proteins or quasi-proteins, that carry out all the biological transformations a cell must perform in order to live, and that control the rate of metabolic processes in an organism. Enzymes, though produced by living organisms, do not require an organic environment: they can function independently, within certain conditional limitations, such as of temperature and acidity.

EPIDEMIOLOGY Literally meaning the study of epidemics, the term epidemiology today applies to any investigation into the causes and course of any disease that affects large numbers of people.

EPITHELIAL CELL A cell that is part of a covering layer or a lining layer, such as on surfaces of cells, cavities, tissues, organs, and vessels of the body.

EPSTEIN-BARR VIRUS A DNA virus (containing only molecules of DNA wrapped in a protein coat) of the family known as herpes viruses; known to be the causal agent of infectious mononucleosis, and causally linked to certain malignancies, such as Burkitt's lymphoma.

ERYTHROCYTE Scientific term for red blood cell; the mature form has no nucleus, is disc-shaped, and gets its red color from its content of hemoglobin, the protein pigment vital to the cell's binding with oxygen; erythrocytes are responsible for the delivery of oxygen to tissues throughout the body.

ERYTHROPOIETIN Hormone produced by the kidneys to stimulate the proliferation and differentiation of red blood cells.

GENES The self-reproducing hereditary units of the cell's chromosomes, genes are made up of sequences of DNA that code for all the proteins needed to build and maintain a living organism; genes contain also noncoding segments that are not yet well understood but may include sequences that play a part in controlling the expression of the gene.

GENE EXPRESSION The process by which a gene's DNA is given the go-ahead by cellular control mechanisms, and transcribes its nucleotide sequences into a strand of RNA. The RNA in turn translates the DNA code, with the aid of enzymes, into the ordered string of amino acids—the end product being a protein.

GENE MAPPING The determination, through various techniques, including inference of the nucleotide sequencing that encodes a known protein product, and direct "reading" of genes' nucleotide sequences, of the locations of different genes or gene units on given chromosomes. Structural genes—those expressed and encoding a protein product—are the easiest to trace and identify: large portions of DNA are "silent," but some of these segments are regulatory in the gene's transcription.

GENETIC CODE The linear arrangement of DNA units along the chromosomes, which scientists have translated into a consistent "formula" base for individuals' protein productions. The translations can predict which amino acid (the unit of proteins) is encoded by three DNA nucleotides in a specific given sequence. Conversely, knowing the sequence of the code allows reasoning from the product to the producer: every amino acid implies its encoding nucleotides.

GENETIC ENGINEERING The process of altering the DNA array of a given cell, through techniques such as cell fusion, cell hybridization or gene splicing, so that the cell can produce more or modified molecules, or encode products completely novel to that cell. Bacteria and yeast are most often used as acceptors of foreign DNA; they can replicate the foreign DNA along with their own, and produce copious amounts of the newly encoded product, such as human interferon, insulin, and growth hormone.

GENE SPLICING   See *Recombinant DNA.*

GLYCOPROTEIN   Proteins with sugar, carbohydrate, and other molecular attachments; complex and large molecules often found on cell surfaces, glycoproteins frequently serve regulatory functions in intercellular communications.

GRAFT-VERSUS-HOST DISEASE (GVHD)   A rejection syndrome in which immune-competent cells or tissue from a donor attack the recipient host's cells or tissues as foreign; such reactions can range from mild and drug-controllable to uncontrollable and fatal.

GRANULOCYTE   A type of white blood cell that differentiates from a myeloid stem cell; in mature form in the blood it responds to antigen-antibody complexes and complement, destroying the targeted material through phagocytosis and enzymatic breakdown.

HEMATOCRIT   Percentage of red blood cells in a given volume of blood.

HEMATOLOGIST   A physician specializing in the treatment of diseases affecting the blood and blood-forming tissues.

HEMOGLOBIN   The oxygen-carrying protein pigment of red blood cells.

HERPES VIRUSES   A family of sturdy viruses (some seventy varieties are known) composed of molecules of DNA wrapped in protein coats. Herpes viruses include those categorized as herpes simplex type 1, usually manifested as cold sores or "fever blisters"; herpes simplex type 2, which usually causes lower-trunk lesions and is responsible for about 80 percent of venereal herpes infections; varicella-zoster virus which causes chicken pox and shingles; Epstein-Barr virus which causes mononucleosis and is linked to several malignancies; and cytomegalovirus, which is a source of fever, hepatitis, and pneumonia-like illness in children and adults.

HISTOCOMPATIBILITY ANTIGENS   The "fingerprints" with which every person's cell surfaces are marked. Controlled by the sixth chromosome, such antigens are inherited markers; they consist of specific proteins common to all of an individual's cells, as well as a set of more exclusive antigens, appearing chiefly on macrophages and B lymphocytes.

HODGKIN'S DISEASE   A proliferation of an abnormal clone of lymphocytes that usually manifests itself in swollen lymph nodes. Treated by irradiation and/or chemotherapy, the disease is now among the most curable of malignancies, with 70 percent of patients surviving five years and longer. The highest incidence of Hodgkin's disease is among persons in their twenties to mid-thirties; some 7,400 persons get the disease each year in the United States.

HOMEOSTASIS Perhaps best described as all cells, all tissues, all organs, and all systems within an organism maintaining structural and functional integrity to assure the continued health and life of the organism; literally, the term means "man staying the same."

HORIZONTAL TRANSMISSION Refers to infectious disease that is spread by contagion or contact, and transmitted by active microorganisms, as distinguished from vertical transmission, which is through altered genes passed on from parent to offspring.

HORMONES Catalytic molecules secreted into the blood by various glands and cells that attach to receptors of different cells and influence their metabolism, either in an inhibitory or stimulatory way.

HUMAN LEUKOCYTE ANTIGENS (HLA) See *Histocompatibility antigens.*

HYBRIDOMA A fused cell whose expressed genes represent both a normal antibody-producing plasma cell and a malignant, prolific version of the plasma cell known as a myeloma cell; hybridomas are used to produce monoclonal antibodies.

HYBRIDS Plants, animals, or even (recently) cells, produced from parents different in kind; current methods of producing hybrid cells involve fusing two cells, so that the expressed genes represent both cells, or inserting genes from one cell into another through gene-splicing techniques.

HYPERTHERMIA Literally meaning high heat, its usage in medical science involves exploiting the difference in the production or absorption of heat among different tissues, or between normal and abnormal (e.g., malignant) tissue, for purposes of diagnosis or treatment. Researchers are investigating the application of heat to cancer patients, in that hyperthermia may selectively damage malignant cells, as compared to normal cells which have better circulation (in tissues) and are better able to dissipate heat.

IMMUNE RESPONSE The bodily recognition of, and reaction against, "nonself" substances, carried out by specialized cells, particularly if the substances invade the deeper tissues of the body or the blood and lymph systems. Immune responses in humans and animals are primarily orchestrated and implemented by the white blood cells.

IMMUNITY An established state of bodily reactivity against particular substances or pathogens. When originally introduced, these substances had activated lymphocytes, and a reservoir of these lymphocytes remains as "memory" cells, to be reactivated if the substances ever appear again.

IMMUNOCOMPETENT Descriptive of white blood cells that respond to regulatory mechanisms as well as to signals for differentiation, activation, and proliferation.

IMMUNOGLOBULINS See *Antibody*.

IMMUNOPROTEINS All the proteins, many of them the products of white blood cells, that play a part in an immune response —such as antibodies and lymphokines. Immunoproteins may stimulate or inhibit a biological step in their own cell line or in other cells.

IMMUNOTHERAPY Any substance or method that is used to elicit a response, or encourage a greater response, to particular antigens (such as those causing disease) by an individual's immune-response system.

INDUCTION THERAPY In relation to cancer, treatment that is intended to bring about a remission, characterized by the absence of, or the greatly reduced number of, detectable malignant cells.

INDUCTIVE EVENT In usages related to cancer causation, the inductive event is the initial blow that renders an individual susceptible to malignant conversion of cells; such events include hereditary or acquired genetic deficiencies or aberrations, an overwhelming invasion by infectious organisms, and a deficiency or retardation in DNA repair.

INTERFERON Traveling molecules, often proteins, formed in response to antigens such as viruses, that bind to other cells and warn them not to accept the foreign genetic material. Interferon is formed in many cells and serves as a chemical signal to other

211

cells to form molecules (probably enzymes) that can break down the foreign genetic material—DNA or RNA—or prevent its transcription into a protein product.

LEUKEMIA A disease of progenitor blood cells, or of cells of one branch of blood cell, resulting in the proliferation of clones of the aberrant cell or cells; frank leukemia occurs when the aberrant cells multiply, become the predominant blood cell, and cannot be eliminated by the individual's immune system.

LEUKOCYTES An inclusive term for all white blood cells, classified as granulocytes, macrophages, monocytes, and lymphocytes.

LYMPH NODES Glands located throughout the lymph system, nodes are way stations and entrapment centers for noxious particles; nodes are often the battlefields where lymphocytes initiate the destructive processes of the immune response against pathogenic invaders.

LYMPH SYSTEM One of two major bodily circulatory systems (the other being the blood system), made up of interconnecting glands and fine vessels, that serves as a processing network for collecting, filtering, and draining waste material. Lymph is an innocuous fluid; and its important traffickers are the lymphocytes, which patrol, and often wage battle, against noxious substances or pathogens that are shunted into the lymph system.

LYMPHOCYTES Small white blood cells that direct and participate in an immune response; highly specialized cells, lymphocytes bear or release molecules that bind to foreign or noxious cells and other substances, and some of them send biological signals to activate other white blood cells.

LYMPHOID STEM CELL See *Stem cell.*

LYMPHOKINES Initially used to designate products of activated lymphocytes, the term now includes all biologically active products of other white blood cells as well. They are regulatory or messenger molecules, often proteins, that stimulate or inhibit processes in recipient cells.

LYMPHOMA A malignancy that arises in the lymph system due to the proliferation of clones of abnormal B lymphocytes; lymphoma is distinguished from B cell leukemias by the tendency of the malignant cells to clump or form tumors in lymphoid tissue, such as lymph nodes and spleen.

MACROPHAGE A large phagocytic white blood cell that serves as a scavenger cell for eliminating broken-down or foreign cells, as well as smaller noxious or foreign particles; macrophages also are secretory cells, producing chemical messages that stimulate or inhibit activity by other cells.

MAINTENANCE THERAPY Drug or irradiation dosages that are given periodically to patients who have attained remission from cancer; maintenance therapy is intended to sustain the remission, and eliminate any lingering malignant cells the patient may harbor.

MAJOR HISTOCOMPATIBILITY COMPLEX (MHC) A sequence of linked genes, found in chromosome 6 in humans, that encodes the self-marking cell proteins known as *histocompatibility antigens* that label cells (and tissues and organs) as "self" or "foreign" for an individual's immune-response system. Closely linked genes in the MHC determine an individual's relative susceptibility to disease and the vigor of cellular interaction in mounting and implementing an immune response.

MALIGNANCY Literally, a tendency to become progressively worse; in medical usage, a malignancy is characterized by cells that are abnormal and nonfunctional, and that exhibit uncontrolled growth and proliferation, often invading tissue and organs that are not an appropriate environment for the malignant cells' normal counterparts.

MEGAKARYOCYTES Large blood cells that remain in the bone marrow and from which platelets are derived; the platelets break off from the megakaryocytes and enter blood circulation.

"MEMORY" CELLS Duplicates, created through division, of B or T lymphocytes that had been activated by particular antigens; such cells are primed to respond and proliferate should their particular antigens ever appear again. Memory cells are central to the action of vaccination and sensitization.

MENDEL'S LAW States the rules by which genetic inheritance operates. Offspring inherit a set of genes from each parent for each trait or characteristic; where the genes differ, those of one parent or the other will be expressed according to the "law." The classic example, set forth by Mendel, holds that if one parent has two genes dictating tallness, which is a dominant trait (**TT**), and the other parent has two genes dictating shortness, which is a recessive trait (ss), then the odds for inheritance by offspring will be: one offspring exhibiting tallness with genes **TT**; two offspring inheriting one gene from each parent (**Ts**), but exhibiting tallness because it is the dominant gene; and one offspring exhibiting shortness with genes ss.

MER Acronym for an extract of the tuberculosis bacillus which is sometimes used in immunotherapy for cancer patients in remission to stimulate immune-system competence.

METABOLISM The physical and chemical processes involved in maintaining life in biological systems, ranging from cells to the organized tissues that constitute a living organism; metabolism is accompanied by transfers of energy.

METABOLITES Nutrients or chemical building blocks that allow a cell to take a biological step in synthesizing a product; often specifically used to indicate components needed to synthesize nucleic acids.

METASTASIS The spread of malignant cells from the originating locale in the body to other sites within the body, usually via the blood and lymph circulatory systems.

MICROORGANISM A tiny living organism, usually meaning one that can be seen only with the use of a microscope; those of medical interest are bacteria, spiral organisms (often called spirochetes), rickettsiae, viruses, molds, and yeasts.

MITOSIS The division of a cell into two identical daughter cells, each of which receives an equal share of chromosomes, cytoplasm, and other cellular structures to allow viable, independent existence.

MOLECULE An organized, functional chemical configuration of atoms; specifically, a unit of two or more atoms that form a definable chemical substance, which, if broken up, changes the substance's character.

MONOCLONAL ANTIBODY An antibody or immunoglobulin (protein) that is attracted to only one particular antigenic chemical configuration, and is synthesized by one particular source cell; the term is now used more specifically to indicate the products of a genetically engineered plasma cell and its clones.

MONOCYTES Small phagocytic white blood cells that circulate in the blood for a few days, then differentiate into the various forms of macrophages.

MULTIPLE MYELOMA A malignancy arising in the bone marrow and caused by proliferating clones of aberrant plasma cells; the disease is often accompanied by copious amounts of unvaried antibodies released into the blood, and the destruction of bone tissue.

MUTANT CELL Any cell which has had its genetic integrity permanently altered, either by internal deletions or rearrangements of gene segments, or by genetic changes induced by external agents such as radiation, chemical carcinogens, or viruses. Mutations are those genetic changes that are transmissible to daughter cells.

MYELOBLAST An undifferentiated blood cell (see *Stem cell*) of the type that gives rise to any of the more mature blood cells with the exception of lymphocytes, and which is preparing for division. The cells of acute leukemia are often blast cells, either myeloblasts or lymphoblasts.

MYELOCYTIC LEUKEMIA See *Acute myelocytic leukemia* and *Chronic myelocytic leukemia.*

MYELOGENOUS LEUKEMIA See *Acute myelocytic leukemia* and *Chronic myelocytic leukemia.*

MYELOID STEM CELL See *Stem cell.*

NATURAL KILLER (NK) CELLS A type of lymphocyte that has not been well characterized, but is believed to account for less than 5 percent of an individual's lymphocytes; NK cells appear to be unique in their ability to kill malignant cells of the host, other individuals, and even of other species, without previous contact with malignant cells and without the interactions that typify immune-response sequences.

NEGATIVE FEEDBACK In terms of cellular activity, negative feedback implies that a regulatory signal (such as the release of a protein) is given by a mature cell to inhibit generation by its precursor or stem cells; this process discourages proliferation of a cell line unless stimulatory signals override the inhibitory signal.

NEOPLASM Literally meaning new growth, the term is often used to describe malignantly transformed cells or tumors.

NEURAMINIDASE An enzyme derived from the cholera bacillus; used in one type of immunotherapy to cleave outer acids from cell-surface proteins on leukemic cells, exposing a more antigenic structure for stimulation of the immune system. The "unmasked" cells are then used to vaccinate patients in remission, to induce greater immune sensitivity against leukemic cells, including those that might arise spontaneously.

NUCLEIC ACIDS Long-chain molecules of high molecular weight, nucleic acids are composed of DNA or RNA subunits; DNA is found in the cell's nucleus, in higher organisms, and RNA is found in the nucleus or in the cytoplasm, where it orders protein production.

NUCLEOTIDE The integral unit of nucleic acids, consisting of one of the four bases—adenine, guanine, cytosine, and thymine (with uracil replacing thymine in the case of RNA)—and its attached sugar and phosphate molecules. A sequence of three nucleotide base pairs encodes a particular amino acid in the construction of a protein; this is the basis of the genetic code for cellular productivity.

NUCLEUS The generally spheroid "command center" within a cell, where the chromosomes are located; it is separated from the cytoplasm by a thin membrane.

"NULL" CELLS Grossly immature lymphocytes that may be lymphoid stem cells; these cells do not bear even early differentiation markers that would indicate their developmental pathway as being that of a B cell or a T cell.

ONCOGENE A gene segment or sequence that, when expressed or "turned on" in a cell, encodes a product (usually some type of protein) that transforms the cell into a potential or actual malignant cell; the encoded products of oncogenes can transform normal cells, sometimes even from different species, into malignant ones.

ONCOGENESIS The process of malignant transformation of cells, specifically those that form tumors or "bulk" aggregates.

ONCOLOGIST A scientist or medical practitioner who specializes in the study or treatment of tumors and other manifestations of malignancy.

ORGANIC Having to do with living organisms; organic compounds are those based on carbon chains or rings which contain hydrogen, and may also contain oxygen, nitrogen, and various other elements.

PATHOGEN   Any substance that causes disease in a host organism; the term is usually applied to disease-causing microorganisms.

PEPTIDE   A short protein. While average proteins are made up of chains several hundred amino acids in length, peptides range from chains only several amino acids long to those that are close in length to average proteins. Peptides are the first abundant end products encoded by genes, and include peptide hormones, enzymes, and antibodies.

PHAGOCYTES   Cells that ingest (and often digest, with the aid of internal enzymes) microorganisms, other cells, and chemical configurations perceived as debris or foreign ("not self"). Phagocytic white blood cells include granulocytes, monocytes, and blood macrophages.

PHILADELPHIA CHROMOSOME   A chromosomal abnormality in which a portion of chromosome 22 has broken off and reattached itself to another chromosome, most often chromosome 9 but sometimes others; this abnormality is highly specific in the recognition of chronic myelocytic leukemia.

PLASMA CELL   A B lymphocyte in its activated and fully differentiated stage. A plasma cell can secrete and release quantities of one particular antibody that is attracted to a specific chemical configuration—its antigen.

PLASMID   A small ring of DNA that is not part of a chromosome, discovered in bacteria. Plasmids are replicated along with the chromosomal DNA in a bacterium (and were probably "donated" by a virus); they are used as vehicles in gene-splicing applications, because they are acceptors of foreign DNA.

PLATELETS   Small discs from the bone marrow cells known as megakaryocytes, that break off and enter blood circulation; platelets are instrumental in normal coagulation of the blood, and in preventing abnormal bleeding.

PLURIPOTENT STEM CELL   See *Stem cell.*

POSITIVE FEEDBACK   In terms of cellular activity, positive feedback implies that a regulatory signal (such as the release of a protein) is given by a mature cell to encourage or stimulate proliferation by its precursor or stem cells; white blood cells that are engaged in fighting infections or other bodily threats send such messages into the bloodstream to initiate the generation of more of their own kind.

PRECURSOR CELL A cell that, along with its daughter cells, can become more developmentally capable or differentiated; examples are the blood stem cells.

PRIMARY RESPONSE With reference to the immune-response system, the primary response indicates initial reactivity to the presence of antigen; it is characterized by the activation of B cells, the differentiation of some of them into antibody-producing plasma cells, the formation of antigen-antibody complexes, and the attraction of complement and granulocytes.

PROGENITOR STEM CELL See *Stem cell.*

PROGNOSIS A forecast as to the probable outcome of a case of a particular disease being treated in a particular way; a prognosis is usually given by the physician to the patient to indicate the patient's prospects for recovery or survival.

PROMOTIONAL EVENT In the two-step theory of cancer causation, there is an initial, predisposing (inductive) event, such as inherited or acquired DNA abnormality. The second event, which may occur days or years later, is called the promotional event (such as cellular disruption by viruses or chemical carcinogens), and stamps the susceptible cells with true malignant potential.

PROSTAGLANDINS A group of about a dozen hormonelike compounds that can be produced as needed by cell membranes in virtually every body tissue; they are potent and are not stored in the body. Prostaglandins are sent out as messengers to other cells, and various ones can induce inflammatory reactions; alter blood pressure; regulate muscle activity and glandular secretions; control the transmission of nerve impulses; defend against infections; and, some scientists believe, defend against malignant cells.

PROTEINS Long chains of amino acids, proteins are the complex end products encoded by genes or cooperative gene sequences (often with a number of different enzyme assists); they are the primary functional and structural components of cells and entire organisms. They may be combined with other molecules, such as carbohydrates and fats.

PROTOCOL In medical practice, a prescribed treatment, based on experience with the disease and customized as much as possible according to type and extent of disease and other patient characteristics. Protocols are sometimes assigned experimentally (from among treatments of proven benefit) to learn which available treatments (such as a new drug or modified combinations of drugs) yield the best results for patients within any given category.

RADIOTHERAPY Treatment with the emissions of any of various forms of radioactive substances, such as X-rays or cobalt; such treatment is intended to destroy cells within the width and depth of focus, when the radioactive substance is beamed from an instrument; or within particular tissues, when implanted in the form of pellets.

RECEPTORS In relation to cells, receptors are surface structures that probably lead into the cytoplasm, and that externally bind specific molecules, such as hormones, complement, antibodies, and other "messenger" molecules released by other cells; the binding signals activation or inhibition of a biological step within the recipient cell.

RECOMBINANT DNA The term describes a process that includes removal of DNA from one host, splicing it into a vehicle (such as an RNA virus or a plasmid) that can successfully donate genes to the intended host, and the acceptance, replication, and expression of the foreign DNA in the new host—often a bacterium, and sometimes yeast or a cell that grows well in tissue culture.

RED BLOOD CELL See *Erythrocyte.*

REGULATORY GENE A gene whose expression does not order the partial or total construction of a protein (as do the so-called "structural genes"), but acts as an on-or-off switch, or a rate-controlling switch, for the expression of other genes, believed to be nearby or adjacent.

REINFORCEMENT THERAPY The periodic (every month, every few months) administration, in patients who are in remission, of the potent drugs and dosages used to induce remission; given in some protocols throughout the maintenance period, alternately with maintenance (less toxic) chemotherapy.

REMISSION Apparent disease-free condition brought about by anti-cancer therapy, that may extend to actual cure. A remission is considered *complete* when there are no leukemic cells in the bone marrow, and other blood cell proportions in the marrow are adequate and normal; a *partial* remission designates a state in which the patient has less than 25 percent of blast cells among the cellular components of the marrow.

REPLICATION Self-duplication; it is the process followed in DNA synthesis in which the double strands of DNA unwind and each strand orders the construction of a new strand identical to its previous complementary strand.

RESCUE THERAPY The follow-up use of antidote drugs or other techniques, such as bone marrow transplants, after the administration of otherwise lethal dosages of drugs or irradiation performed in an effort to totally eradicate malignant cells. Rescue therapy either revives normal cells or induces the regeneration of normal cells, following the aggressive anti-cancer treatment.

RESTRICTION ENZYMES Enzymes, obtained from bacteria, that can recognize and cleave short nucleotide sequences that flank encoding gene segments and can thus cut up and destroy invading DNA. Restriction enzymes are used in the laboratory to snip portions of DNA into gene-sized pieces, for purposes of examination or gene-splicing applications.

RETINOIDS Synthetic analogues of vitamin A, this class of drugs is being investigated for possible refinement into cancer preventives; several forms have been found to convert, in the laboratory, leukemic cells into differentiated and mature cells.

REVERSE TRANSCRIPTASE An enzyme discovered in RNA viruses; the enzyme's action enables a strand of RNA in a host cell to dictate the synthesis of a corresponding strand of DNA (the reverse of the usual transcription pattern), thus ensuring transmission of the genetic message in heritable form to future generations of the invaded host cell.

RNA Molecules of ribonucleic acid existing as a single strand; found in the cell's nucleus or cytoplasm, RNA assists in translating the genetic message of DNA into the production of proteins.

RNA TUMOR VIRUS A variety of virus that can cause malignancies, including leukemia, in various species of animals; its mode of action is to use a special enzyme (reverse transcriptase, defined above) to integrate its RNA message into a host cell's DNA. Through the revised DNA message (mutation) and its encoded protein product, the cell is transformed into a malignant one.

SECONDARY RESPONSE With reference to the immune-response system, the secondary response indicates delayed re-activity to the presence of antigen; it is characterized by the activation of T cells and macrophages.

SENSITIZATION The process by which the immune-response system becomes "aware" of certain antigens; sensitization involves exposure to the antigen, and usually implies, when it is successful, specifically reactive responses by T cells in addition to the activation of B cells and the production of antibodies.

SERUM Literally, the clear portion of any animal liquid separated from its more solid elements; usually used to refer to the clear liquid of the blood (also called plasma) separated from blood cells, platelets, and fibrinogen (coagulation proteins).

SIALIC ACID Silicone-based compound attached to the surface of glycoproteins on cell surfaces; removal of this via enzyme cleavage is intended to expose antigenic structures on leukemia cells, and such modified cells are used for vaccination of leukemia patients in one type of immunotherapy.

SPLEEN A glandlike organ, about five or six inches in length, located in the upper left abdomen, and surrounded by the stomach, the diaphragm, the left lung, and kidney. The spleen generates a small percentage of blood cells, and is a way station for white blood cells, particularly lymphocytes and macrophages.

STEM CELL A cell that is the progenitor of a particular line (or lines) of daughter cells that evolve into more specialized cells. With reference to blood cells, a *pluripotent stem cell* is one that may give rise to any type or pathway of blood cell development; a *lymphoid stem cell* gives rise to any of the types of lymphocyte; a *myeloid stem cell* can give rise to red blood cells, megakaryocytes, granulocytes, monocytes, and macrophages; and a *unipotent stem cell* is an intermediate-stage progenitor that can give rise to only one type of blood cell, such as granulocytes or red blood cells.

STEROIDS Literally, a group of compounds that resemble cholesterol chemically; generally used in medicine to indicate hormones of this chemical family, such as those produced by the adrenal glands, used to treat lymphocytic leukemia because they suppress the growth of lymphocytes.

SYNTHESIS Although the term literally means the artificial building-up of a chemical compound by assembly of its elements, synthesis is also used to indicate the natural assembly of a product by an organic entity; for example, a plasma cell synthesizes antibody.

SYSTEMIC   Not confined to a particular bodily site, but ranging through interdependent or interconnected parts; used in reference to disease, "systemic" usually indicates that the pathological process affects the body as a whole, such as when malignant cells are in the circulatory systems.

T CELLS   A type of lymphocyte that originates in the bone marrow but spends its formative period in the thymus gland before entering circulation. T cells are critical regulators and orchestrators of effective immune responses, particularly against larger antigens such as foreign or aberrant cells; T cells interact instructively with other white blood cells.

TEMPLATE   A pattern or mold; in terms of genetic activity, for example, an expressed segment of DNA is said to serve as a template for the construction of a strand of RNA; the RNA acts as an executor in seeing the DNA message translated into a finished protein or protein segment.

THYMIC HORMONES   Regulatory molecules produced by cells in the thymus gland that appear to have a strong maturational influence on undeveloped T cells during their formative period in the thymus.

THYMOCYTE   A precursor or immature T cell.

THYMUS   A gland in the lower neck, beneath the thyroid gland; the thymus shrinks to a vestige by adolescence, and is essentially a mass of lymphocytes. Precursor T cells spend a formative period in the thymus, influenced there by hormones that appear to be released by epithelial cells lining the thymus.

TISSUE CULTURE   The isolation of particular cells in laboratory dishes, where they are supplied any nutrients or other chemicals that will encourage them to grow and synthesize their genetically ordered products. These products are then examined for any that are not normally produced by such cells, that are missing, or that are abnormal variations of usual products. These deviations indicate the presence of foreign (e.g., viral), defective, or mutant genetic activity.

TRANSFORMATION   Literally, change or conversion of form or structure; used with reference to malignant cells, transformation implies conversion of cells to a status outside of the normal cellular and bodily controls, particularly with regard to division and proliferation.

TRANSPLANTATION ANTIGENS See *Histocompatibility antigens.*

TUMOR An aggregation of malignant cells, or any new tissue that persists and grows independently of its surrounding structures, and serves no functional purpose.

ULTRASOUND Sound waves that vibrate at extremely high frequencies. Ultrasound technology is often used diagnostically in medical practice: the differences in "bounce-back" pattern distinguishes normal from abnormal responses in tissues. Ultrasound is being used experimentally as a potentiator of chemotherapy, in that it may make cells more permeable to drugs.

VACCINE A solution containing part of, or an altered form of, an infectious microorganism against which protection is desired; the vaccine is not dangerous in itself (e.g., the microbe is dead, or only part of its coat is used), but is intended to "introduce" the microbe to the vaccinated person's immune-response system, so that if a live or whole version of the microbe ever appears, it will be destroyed by a primed immune system.

VARICELLA-ZOSTER A type of herpes virus that is the causative agent of chicken pox and shingles, and which can pose life-threatening infections in patients whose immune system is suppressed due to chemotherapy.

VERTICAL TRANSMISSION With reference to cell mutations caused by viruses, vertical transmission describes the persistence of cellular mutation through the genes, passed on from parent to offspring, usually for generations.

VIROLOGIST A scientist or medical scientist who specializes in the study of viruses and/or the diagnosis or treatment of viral diseases.

VIRUS A microscopic, infectious parasite whose varieties infect plants, animals, humans, and even bacteria; viruses consist of segments of either DNA or RNA, and are of varying sizes and genetic complexity. Their outer wrapping is a protein coat with protruding protein spikes, which serve as entry mechanisms (like hyperdermic needles) for invading cells.

WHITE BLOOD CELLS   Collectively called leukocytes, white blood cells include lymphocytes, granulocytes, monocytes, and macrophages—and the precursor cells of these lines.

X-RAY   Electromagnetic waves similar to light, but of a much shorter wavelength; a kind of radiation that can penetrate the human body and be used for illuminating portions of it (as in X-ray films or plates), or, at higher voltages, to irradiate portions of the body intended to be destroyed.

SOURCES OF HELP
AND INFORMATION

In this section we describe or list sources of information, financial aid, or other services for leukemia patients and their families, and books and other printed materials about leukemia and leukemia patients, that we believe to be reliable, helpful, readily available, and accessible. Particular communities or medical centers may offer, in addition, local services or resources that are beyond the scope of our research or knowledge.

On the local level, we recommend that you direct your inquiries about possible additional help to the nearest unit or branch of the American Cancer Society or the Leukemia Society of America, because of these agencies' extensive national network. Current information and referral services are offered also through a national network of Cancer Information Service Offices, cooperatively sponsored by the National Cancer Institute and the American Cancer Society. Information is given over the phone and callers need not give their names (see Table 3).

The addresses of all agencies and organizations referred to in this section appear on page 234.

TABLE 3. CANCER INFORMATION
SERVICE OFFICES

CALIFORNIA
LAC-USC Cancer Center
From Area Codes (213), (714)
and (805): 1-800-252-9066
Rest of California: (213)
226-2374

COLORADO
Colorado Regional Cancer
Center
1-800-332-1850

TABLE 3. (Continued)

CONNECTICUT
Yale University
Comprehensive Cancer Center
1-800-922-0824

DELAWARE
Fox Chase Cancer Center
1-800-523-3586

DISTRICT OF COLUMBIA
(Includes suburban Maryland
and Northern Virginia)
Cancer Communications for
Metropolitan Washington
(202) 232-2833

FLORIDA
Comprehensive Cancer Center
for the State of Florida
Florida: 1-800-432-5953
Dade County: (305) 547-6920

HAWAII
Cancer Information Line
Oahu: 536-0111
Neighbor Islands: Ask operator
for Enterprise 6702

ILLINOIS
Illinois Cancer Council
Illinois: 1-800-972-0586
Chicago: (312) 346-9813

MAINE
Maine Cancer Information
Service
1-800-225-7034

MARYLAND
The Johns Hopkins Oncology
Center
1-800-492-1444

MASSACHUSETTS
Massachusetts Cancer
Information Service
1-800-952-7420

MINNESOTA
Minnesota Cancer Council
1-800-582-5262

MONTANA
Montana Cancer Information
Service
1-800-525-0231

NEW HAMPSHIRE
New Hampshire Cancer
Information Service
1-800-225-7034

NEW JERSEY
Fox Chase Cancer Center
1-800-523-3586

NEW MEXICO
New Mexico Cancer
Information Service
1-800-525-0231

NEW YORK
Roswell Park Memorial Institute
New York State:
1-800-462-7255
Erie County: (716) 845-4400

NEW YORK CITY
Memorial Sloan-Kettering
Cancer Center
(212) 794-7982

NORTH CAROLINA
Duke Comprehensive Cancer
Center
North Carolina: 1-800-672-0943
Durham County: (919)
286-2266

TABLE 3. *(Continued)*

PENNSYLVANIA
Fox Chase Cancer Center
1-800-822-3963

TEXAS
M.D. Anderson Hospital
and Tumor Institute
Texas: 1-800-392-2040
Houston: (713) 792-3245

VERMONT
Vermont Cancer Information
Service
1-800-225-7034

WASHINGTON
Fred Hutchinson Cancer
Research Center
1-800-552-7212

WISCONSIN
Wisconsin Clinical Cancer Center
University of Wisconsin
1-800-362-8038

WYOMING
Wyoming Cancer Information
Service
1-800-525-0231

TREATMENT FACILITIES

Medical centers that offer state of the art capability in leukemia treatment, as recognized by the National Cancer Institute, are listed, alphabetically by state, below. (Also see chapter 4, "Optimal Treatment Centers.")

Comprehensive Cancer Center
University of Alabama at
   Birmingham
Birmingham, AL 35294

University of Arizona Cancer
   Center
Tucson, AZ 85721

University of California at
   San Diego
La Jolla, CA 92093

Kenneth Norris Jr. Cancer
   Research Institute
University of Southern
   California
Los Angeles, CA 90033

UCLA Jonsson Comprehensive
   Cancer Center
UCLA School of Medicine
Los Angeles, CA 90024

Northern California Cancer
   Program
Palo Alto, CA 94305

Colorado Regional Cancer
   Center, Inc.
Denver, CO 80206

Yale University Comprehensive
   Cancer Center
New Haven, CT 06510

Georgetown University/
  Howard University
  Comprehensive Cancer Center
Washington, DC 20007

Comprehensive Cancer Center
  for the State of Florida
University of Miami School of
  Medicine/Jackson Memorial
  Medical Center
Miami, FL 33134

Cancer Center of Hawaii
University of Hawaii at Manoa
Honolulu, HI 96822

Northwestern University Cancer
  Center
Evanston, IL 60201

University of Chicago Cancer
  Research Center
Chicago, IL 60637

Ephraim McDowell Community
  Cancer Network, Inc.
Lexington, KY 40506

Johns Hopkins Oncology Center
Baltimore, MD 21205

National Cancer Institute
Clinical Center
Bethesda, MD 21609

Sidney Farber Cancer Institute
Boston, MA 02115

Hubert H. Humphrey Cancer
  Research Center
Boston University School of
  Medicine
Boston, MA 02215

Cancer Center, Tufts-New
  England Medical Center
Medford, MA 02155

Comprehensive Cancer Center
  of Metropolitan Detroit
Detroit, MI 48201

Mayo Comprehensive Cancer
  Center
Rochester, MN 55901

Norris Cotton Cancer Center
Dartmouth-Hitchcock Medical
  Center
Hanover, NH 03755

Cancer Research and Treatment
  Center
University of New Mexico
Albuquerque, NM 87131

Cancer Research Center
Albert Einstein College of
  Medicine
Bronx, NY 10461

Roswell Park Memorial Institute
Buffalo, NY 14203

Sloan-Kettering Institute for
  Cancer Research/Memorial
  Sloan-Kettering Cancer
  Center
New York, NY 10021

Hospital for Joint Diseases and
  Medical Center
New York, NY 10035

Mount Sinai Medical Center
New York, NY 10029

New York University Medical
  Center
New York, NY 10016

Columbia University Cancer
  Research Center
College of Physicians &
  Surgeons
New York, NY 10032

University of Rochester Cancer
    Center
Rochester, NY 14627

Comprehensive Cancer Center
Duke University Medical Center
Durham, NC 27710

Cancer Research Center,
    University of North Carolina
Chapel Hill, NC 27514

Oncology Research Center
Bowman-Gray School of
    Medicine
Winston-Salem, NC 27103

The Ohio State University
    Comprehensive Cancer Center
Columbus, OH 43210

University of Pennsylvania
    Comprehensive Cancer Center
(Includes Institute for Cancer
    Research, Fox Chase, PA)
Philadelphia, PA 19111

Puerto Rico Cancer Center
University of Puerto Rico,
    Medical Sciences Campus
San Juan, PR 00931

Roger Williams General Hospital
Providence, RI 02908

Memphis Regional Cancer
    Center
University of Tennessee
Memphis, TN 38163

St. Jude Children's Research
    Hospital
Memphis, TN 38101

The University of Texas
    Medical Branch Hospitals
Galveston, TX 77550

The University of Texas System
    Cancer Center
M.D. Anderson Hospital and
    Tumor Institute
Houston, TX 77030

Vermont Regional Cancer
    Center
University of Vermont
Burlington, VT 05405

Medical College of Virginia
    Cancer Center
Richmond, VA 23219

Fred Hutchinson Cancer
    Research Center
Seattle, WA 98104

The University of Wisconsin
    Clinical Cancer Center
Madison, WI 53706

Milwaukee Children's Hospital
Milwaukee, WI 53233

FINANCIAL ASSISTANCE

1. Outpatients being treated for leukemia may obtain from the
Leukemia Society of America about $750 per year to help pay for
drugs, blood-processing costs related to transfusions, transporta-

tion to and from the doctor's office or medical center for treatments, and X-ray therapy (not diagnostic). This aid is provided through application to the Society's state chapters. Check local directories under Leukemia Society of America; if there is no listing write or call the national headquarters for referral to the nearest branch office.

2. The possibilities of financial aid from state or local funds, organizations or agencies should be checked through regional offices of the Cancer Information Service.

3. Financial assistance to help meet the costs of homemaker-home health aide services for caring for patients with advanced cancer at home is provided by Cancer Care, Inc. This agency currently provides services chiefly in the region of New York, New Jersey, and Connecticut.

4. Some of the major cancer treatment centers have funding to help support or to carry entirely the costs of treatment to patients who are entered in protocols of investigational treatment (see chapter 3). Check with the prospective or chosen institution to see if such funding is available, and whether or not the particular patient qualifies.

COUNSELING

1. Cancer Information Service Offices, affiliated with cancer treatment centers, the National Cancer Institute, and the American Cancer Society offer information and referral service over the telephone. Check Table 3 for the office serving your area.

These information centers provide data on causes, detection, diagnosis, and treatment of cancer; medical facilities in the region served; and can recommend local resources for rehabilitation programs, home-care assistance, financial aid, and emotional counseling. They provide quick phone responses, and will also send printed materials upon request.

2. State and city chapters of the Leukemia Society of America refer callers to local services and sources of emotional support.

3. The American Cancer Society, headquartered in New York City, has some sixty state and large-city divisions, some 3,000 county-level units, and almost 2,000 community-level branches.

Trained volunteers in *unit* offices can provide information and refer callers to local services and resources.

4. Group and individual counseling, by professional and social workers, for advanced cancer patients and family members who are coping with home-care as well as emotional or economic difficulties, is provided by Cancer Care, Inc., headquartered in New York City. Primarily serving the tri-state area of New York, New Jersey, and Connecticut, this agency provides counseling at its offices in this region. However, the agency responds to telephone requests for assistance from any part of the country.

OTHER DIRECT SERVICES

1. American Cancer Society units (affiliate offices providing services at the county level) offer guidance and a number of services to cancer patients at home. Although resources vary around the country, most units can provide: (1) sickroom supplies, personal comfort items, surgical dressings, and the loan of larger equipment such as hospital beds and wheelchairs; (2) transportation to and from the doctor's office or the medical center for treatments; (3) help with health care at home, through visits by ACS's own volunteers.

ACS divisions (state-level offices) participate in blood-donor recruitment programs; and may assist cancer patients by "enrolling" them as blood clients, without obliging the patient to pay for blood or solicit replacement donors for transfusions.

2. In small towns and rural areas, state, county, or city public health departments often can send nurses or other health aides to guide family members in providing health care for cancer patients at home. Visits are free of charge. Depending on local circumstances, these departments may be able to provide sickroom supplies and loans of larger equipment, such as patient hoists, hospital beds, and wheelchairs.

PLACES TO STAY: SPECIAL CONSIDERATION

1. Ronald McDonald Houses are reasonably priced (e.g., $8 per night in Boston) residences in cities where major cancer treatment centers are located; they are geared to accommodate out-of-town parents whose children are undergoing treatment at the medical centers. Most of the residences provide extras such as laundry facilities, kitchen and dining facilities, and play areas; child patients often can join the parents at the residence during "off-hours" from treatment schedules.

Ronald McDonald Houses are supported financially by fund-raising efforts spearheaded by the Ronald McDonald Foundation in Oak Brook, Illinois and franchise restaurants of the McDonald chain; with additional contributions for local residences coming from other local businesses, corporations, and individuals. Each residence is administered locally by nonprofit corporations set up for the purpose; directors usually include physicians affiliated with the local cancer treatment centers.

As of mid-1983, Ronald Houses are operational in some thirty cities; and, reportedly, sponsoring groups in some thirty-odd additional cities are in the development stages of opening Ronald McDonald Houses. Check the telephone listings under "Ronald McDonald House" in any given city.

2. Some medical centers have rooms or apartments available for families of out-of-town patients, in staff housing complexes on or nearby the medical center grounds. In some of the large medical centers specializing in the treatment of childhood cancer, a parent can room in, sharing the child's hospital room or an adjoining room. Call the prospective institution's patient services department, patient ombudsman, or public relations department.

TRANSPORTATION: SPECIAL CONSIDERATION

1. Depending on schedules and commitments, military plane transportation can sometimes be arranged (free of charge) to meet the needs of cancer patients and their families, such as for emergency treatment at a distant medical center or for visitation by family members. The Air National Guard can be contacted on the

state level; on the federal level, the United States Air Force or the United States Army can be contacted at the nearest installation, if known, or by calling telephone directory-assistance operators in the state's capital city.

2. The American Cancer Society began a program in late 1981 to establish liaisons with corporations who maintain corporate planes for cross-country or regional transportation for company personnel; such business flights are often not fully booked, and if destinations coincide with those of cancer patients (and their families) needing transportation to or from medical centers, free hitches may be possible. Some corporations even arrange for detours to accommodate patients, or make special nonscheduled flights. IBM and American Express have already signed on, with Connecticut and Westchester, New York, divisions of ACS, for the Corporate Angel Network (CAN), and other corporations are following suit. Check your nearest ACS division for prospects in your area.

NATIONAL ORGANIZATIONS FOR PATIENTS AND FAMILIES

1. Make Today Count is a guidance and support organization for cancer patients and other seriously ill patients, with chapters in over 100 cities. Chapters frequently invite health-care professionals and psychological counselors to attend their meetings. The group emphasizes the mutual growth of patients and family members in understanding the effects of life-threatening illness, and in dealing with their real needs and fears. New members receive guidance in expanding personal and outside resources, and are helped to develop their own ways of coping.

2. The Candlelighters is an organization with over 150 chapters for parents who have or have had children with cancer. Some groups have youth auxiliaries for teenage cancer patients and teenage siblings of children with cancer. Chapters sponsor twenty-four-hour crisis phone-lines, professional counseling, meetings, information services (e.g., newsletters, handbooks of local resources), and self-help groups; members often help each other with babysitting, transportation, wig banks, and hospital visiting.

The executive arm of the parent's chapters is The Candlelighters Foundation, which helps new groups form and issues a variety of publications, including an annual progress report which summarizes current treatment results and research in childhood cancers; the reports are written in nontechnical language by physicians specializing in cancer treatment.

3. CHUMS is the acronym for Cancer Hopefuls United for Mutual Support, an organization formed in 1981 to combat the discrimination and prejudice against cancer patients. CHUMS also arranges forums where members can question cancer specialists, as well as self-help meetings for members. CHUMS is headquartered in New York City, where it has several hundred members. It has regional representatives, all of whom are professional psychological counselors with a history of cancer, in forty states.

NATIONAL HEADQUARTERS OF AGENCIES AND ORGANIZATIONS

American Cancer Society, Public Information Office, 777 Third Avenue, New York, NY 10017. (212) 736-3030.

Cancer Care, Inc., One Park Avenue, New York, NY 10016. (212) 679-5700.

Cancer Information Service, national toll-free line, (800) 638-6694. See listing of service offices, Table 3.

Candlelighters Foundation, Suite 1011, 2025 Eye Street, N.W., Washington, DC 20006. (202) 659-5136.

CHUMS, 3310 Rochambeau Avenue, Bronx, NY 10467. (212) 655-7566.

Leukemia Society of America, 800 Second Avenue, New York, NY 10017. (212) 573-8484.

Make Today Count, 218 South Sixth Street, Burlington, IA 52601. (319) 753-6521.

National Cancer Institute (for publications), Office of Cancer Communications, National Cancer Institute, Bethesda, MD 20205. Public Information Office: (301) 496-5583.

FURTHER READING

The sources listed below range from brochures and booklets to workbooks and books. The descriptions are meant to suggest their helpfulness, relevance, or possible interest for individual readers. Addresses of agencies and organizations are on page 234.

PAMPHLETS ABOUT OR RELATED TO LEUKEMIA

Single copies available free from the National Cancer Institute:

Chemotherapy and You—a guide to what to expect during treatment; how to deal with unpleasant side-effects; and what serious side-effects should be reported to the physician.

Radiotherapy and You—a guide to self-help during and after treatments; and common side effects and how to handle them.

What You Need to Know About Adult Leukemia—facts about leukemia, including how it is diagnosed and treated; brief discussions of emotional aspects and research.

What You Need to Know About Childhood Leukemia—same format as pamphlet about adult leukemia. Also available in Spanish.

Eating Hints and *Diet and Nutrition*—advice on coping with loss of appetite and other eating problems experienced by adult and child cancer patients.

The Leukemic Child—Written by a newspaper feature writer, Mikie Sherman, the mother of a young child who died of acute lymphocytic leukemia, this eighty-page booklet talks to other parents about the disease itself, emotional and practical aspects of dealing with hospitalization of a young child and the child's return home.

Available free from the American Cancer Society:

Facts on Leukemia—a pamphlet about leukemia—risk factors, signs and symptoms, diagnosis, treatment, prognosis, and care during remission.

Parents' Handbook on Leukemia—written by staff members of the Pediatric Oncology Clinic at Rhode Island Hospital, this sixty-page booklet describes the leukemic process, the operation of a cancer clinic, medications and drug actions, common health questions, and parental roles.

Available free from the Leukemia Society of America:

What Everyone Should Know About Leukemia—information about the major types of leukemia, causal and risk factors, symptoms, diagnosis, treatments, and research approaches.

Leukemia, the Nature of the Disease—a discussion of the cellular changes and systemic effects of leukemia; includes pictures of slides of magnified normal and leukemic blood samples, and normal and leukemic bone marrow and lymph node specimens.

Emotional Aspects of Childhood Leukemia—a handbook for parents to help guide themselves and their children through the emotional aspects of diagnosis and treatment; offers some help with handling the possibility of death.

UPDATES ON LEUKEMIA RESEARCH AND STATISTICS

(single copies available free)

American Cancer Society *Facts and Figures*—an annual report on incidence, prevalence, and survival rates for various types of cancer, including leukemia; a brief description of the services of the Society.

Leukemia Society of America *Annual Report*—brief description of the services and membership of the Society; abstracts of research projects (over 100) receiving funding from the Society.

National Cancer Institute *Research Report: Progress Against Leukemia*—categorized (e.g., virology, immunology) presentation of research advances into the causation of leukemia and treatment; revised periodically.

Two other NCI *Research Reports* may be of interest: *Drugs vs. Cancer* and *Virus-Cancer Research*. Both pamphlets are written in categorized, narrative style understandable to the layman; they describe respectively, the various drugs used in chemotherapy and increased survival rates with newer types of drugs; and the possible roles of viruses in cancer causation. Revised periodically.

Candlelighters Foundation *Progress Reports*—annual journal on current treatments and research related to childhood cancer, with particular emphasis on leukemia; topic summaries (e.g., "Progress after Relapse of Acute Leukemia," "Marrow Transplantation for Acute Leukemia") are written in nontechnical language by physicians specializing in cancer treatment.

Books for Children with Cancer

You and Leukemia: A Day at a Time by Lynn S. Baker (New York: W. B. Saunders Publishing Co., 1978), $7.95. Magazine-size and some 200 pages, this handbook was originally developed by staff members at the Mayo Comprehensive Cancer Center in Rochester, Minnesota for youngsters who are being treated for leukemia. Recommended for those eight years of age or older (too childish for teenagers). Describes the body and cellular life, the leukemic process, living with leukemia, and treatments (in considerable detail). Very thorough, with no punches pulled. Glossary; amply illustrated.

Hospital Days, Treatment Ways. A coloring book for young children with cancer, illustrating hospital personnel, procedures, and treatments. Available free from the National Cancer Institute.

PERSONAL ACCOUNTS ABOUT COPING WITH CANCER

Angela Ambrosia by Ray Errol Fox (New York: Alfred A. Knopf, 1979), $7.95. "Trying to grow up in a bizarre and constricted world," Angela had been living with chronic myelocytic leukemia for ten years. The author, a filmwriter chosen by Angela to tell her story, brings an immediacy to her fright, fight, and ordinary experiences; and to her relationships with doctors, fellow patients, and family from her teenage years into her mid-twenties.

Eric by Doris Lund (New York: Dell Publishing Co., 1974), $1.75. The story of a seventeen-year-old boy with acute leukemia, written by his mother; tells how patient and parent cope and express love.

How Could I Not Be Among You? by Ted Rosenthal (New York: Avon Books, 1973), $1.50. A first-person account, in prose, poetry, and photographs, of the thoughts, fears, values, and philosophy of a thirty-one-year-old man with acute leukemia.

Learning to Live with Cancer by Kelly M. Sveinson (New York: St. Martin's, 1977), $7.95. Written by a middle-aged Canadian businessman who was diagnosed as having Hodgkin's disease in 1962, this personal account, strong on pragmatism, provides formulas to help cancer patients "seize the day."

Shannon: A Book for Parents of Children with Leukemia by Leonard F. Johnson and Marc Miller (New York: Hawthorn Books, 1975), $6.95. An account of a young girl, Shannon, with acute leukemia, written by her physician and her grandfather; describes the disease itself and how the patient, her family, and medical personnel deal with the disease, both pragmatically and emotionally.

Stay of Execution: A Sort Of Memoir by Stewart Alsop (Philadelphia–New York: J. B. Lippincott Co., 1973), $9.95. A well-known political reporter and columnist (*Newsweek*) describes the emotional and practical aspects of dealing with a condition diagnosed as "preleukemia" for two years. He also talks about his family and career; famous people he knew; and his values, fears, and thoughts of death.

INDEX

aclacinomycin, 187
acute granulocytic leukemia. *See*
    acute myelocytic leukemia
acute lymphatic leukemia, 80
acute lymphocytic leukemia, 17
    clustering of cases of, 72
    incidence of, 19, 20
    MHC antigen on cells of patients
      with, 154
    prognosis for chemotherapy in
      children with, 193–94
    radiotherapy and, 107–8
    treatment of, 20
acute myelocytic leukemia, 17
    family studies, 40–41
    incidence, 20
    induced, 70
    prognosis for chemotherapy in
      adults with, 194–95
    vaccination studies in, 178–80
Acyclovir, 196
adult leukemia patients
    care of, 141–46
    emotional reactions of, 142–46
    handling side effects of therapy
      in, 144
    most common leukemia types in,
      20–21
    psychotherapy for, 146
    sexual problems of, 143
    use of drugs by, 144–46
age
    acute lymphocytic leukemia
      incidence and, 20, 21
    allogenic bone marrow transplants
      and, 112
    chemotherapy and, 81

Hodgkin's disease and, 23
    leukemia incidence and, 1–2
aging, DNA damage and, 38
aleukemic leukemia, 17
alkylating agents, 86
    DNA mutations and, 97
allogenic bone marrow trans-
    plantation, 109–20
    recipients of, 112
Alsop, Stewart, 141–42, 143
American Cancer Society, 130
    epidemiological study of cancer,
      153–54
    services of, 231
amino acids, 30–33
aminopterin, 85
m-AMSA, 187
amygdalin. *See* Laetrile
analgesics, 144–46
    for leukemic children, 140
anemia
    chemotherapy and, 97–98
    erythrocytes and, 8
animals
    cancer-causing viral mutations
      in, 43–48, 52–53
    drug tests in, 158
ankylosing spondylitis, 66
antibiotics
    anti-leukemia, 87
    DNA mutations and, 96–97
    during chemotherapy, 99
    infections and, 102–4
    side effects of, 105
antibodies
    B-cell secretion of, 14–15
    in children, 72

antibodies (*continued*)
  immune response and, 60–64
  to RNA virus, T-cell leukemia
    and, 53
antigens
  complement and, 13
  defined, 58–59
  hypersensitivity and, 60
  immune response and, 60–64
  leukemic cells and, 67–68
  lymphocyte recognition of
    macrophages and, 13–15
  marrow stem cells and, 7
  See also MHC antigens
anti-leukemia drugs, 85–89, 90–92
  alkylating agents, 86
  antibiotics, 87
  antimetabolites, 86–87
  antiviral agents, 89
  basis for action of, 89–90
  discovery of, 85
  hormones, 87
  mitosis inhibitors, 87–88
  pseudoenzymes, 88
antimetabolites, 86–87
  DNA mutations and, 96–97
antioxidants, 192
antipsychotic drugs, 145
antiviral agents, anti-leukemia, 88
aplastic anemia, leukemia and, 70
appetite, loss of, 144
ataxia telangiectasia, 70
autoimmune diseases, 60, 70
autologous bone marrow transplants,
    119–20
  monoclonal antibodies and, 183

B cells
  antigens and, 58–59
  chronic lymphocytic leukemia
    and, 20, 21
  function of, 14–15
bacteria
  gene-splicing studies, 161–65
  phagocytosis and, 11
  restriction enzymes of, 161–62
  See also pathogens
basic research, 156–60
basophilic leukemia, 17
BCG vaccine, immunotherapy in
    leukemia and, 120–21
biological response modifiers

granulopoietin, 177
  interferons, 171–75
  lithium carbonate, 176–77
  T-cell growth factor and
    macrophage factors, 176
  thymosin, 175–76
  vitamin A derivatives, 176
blood cells
  causes of imbalance in, 5
  cellular components of, 5
  development and activities of,
    5, 7–15
  diagnosis of leukemia and, 23–24
  leukemic cells in marrow and, 16
  lymph fluid and, 5
  Philadelphia chromosome and, 21
  types of, 10
  See also erythrocytes; leukocytes;
    megakaryocytes
blood platelets. *See* platelets
blood system, 6
  functions of, 4–5
  immune responses and, 58
blood tests for leukemic children,
    140–41
blood transfusions
  prior to bone marrow transplan-
    tation, 112
  problems with, 101–5
blood-forming tissues, leukemia
    and, 4
Bloom's syndrome, leukemia and, 70
body chemistry, cell differentiation
    and, 2–3
bone marrow
  blood cell derivation and, 7
  blood cell production of, 5
  chemotherapy and, 94, 97
  diagnosis of leukemia and, 24–25
  induced suppression of, 70
  leukemic cells in, 4, 16, 20
  megakaryocytes in, 8
  in multiple myeloma, 22
  See also stem cells
bone marrow transplants. *See*
    allogenic bone marrow trans-
    plantation; autologous bone
    marrow transplantation
Burkitt's lymphoma, Epstein-Barr
    virus and, 54
butylated hydroxyanisole (BHA),
    192

cancer
    abnormal cell behavior in, 2–3
    biological response modifiers,
        170–77
    early diagnosis of, 154
    epidemiological study of
        causes of, 153–54
    genetic abnormalities and, 40–41
    immune response and, 65
    incidence of, 27
    information service offices,
        115–17
    leukemia as form of, 4
    personal accounts about coping
        with, 237–38
    preventive drugs, 192–93
    proteins and, 35–36
    susceptibility studies, 153–54
    toxic substances and, 41
    viral mutations in animals and,
        43–48
    See also malignant cells; two-step
        theory of cancer
Cancer Care, Inc., 130
"cancer families," 40–41
"cancer genes"
    in animals and humans, 48–52
    research in, 185
    viruses and, 42–55
cancer patients, national organiza-
    tions for, 233–34
Candlelighters, 233–34
carcinogens
    effects of, 41–42
    leukemia and, 76
    See also two-step theory of cancer
cell cycle, antileukemic drugs and,
    86
cell differentiation, 2–3
cell fusion, production of mono-
    clonal antibodies and, 180–81
cell proliferation in chronic
    myelocytic leukemia, 21
cells
    abnormal in cancer, 2–3
    acute lymphocytic leukemia and,
        20
    malignancy-associated markers
        on, 154
    transfer of normal genes into,
        168–69

transformation into leukemic cells,
    28
    viruses and, 42–43
    See also blood cells; defective
        cells; DNA; foreign cells;
        leukemic cells; malignant cells;
        stem cells
central nervous system, radiotherapy
    and, 106, 108
chemotherapy, 83–98
    in acute lymphocytic leukemia, 20
    anti-leukemic drugs used in,
        85–89, 90–92
    basis of, 83–84
    cell phases and, 188
    central nervous system involve-
        ment and, 9
    chronic myelocytic leukemia and,
        21–22
    circadian rhythms and, 189–91
    drug administration routes, 84
    effectiveness of, 93–96
    individual protocols for, 96
    induced DNA mutations and,
        96–97
    marijuana side effects, 145
    objectives of, 78–79
    patient care during, 84–85
    potential use of gene splicing in,
        168
    prediction of response to, 156,
        193–95
    pregnancy and, 98
    protection against viral infections
        and, 195–97
    remissions and relapses after,
        see relapses; remissions
    "resting" leukemic cells and,
        80–81, 93
    side effects of, 96–98
    sterility and, 98
    supportive therapy and, *see*
        supportive therapy
    toxicity and, 93–94
chicken pox
    childhood leukemia patients and,
        104
    protection against, 195–96
childhood asthma, 66
childhood cancer, books on, 237
childhood leukemia
    chemotherapy and, 193–94

childhood leukemia (*continued*)
  "clustering," 72
  emotional reaction to, 125–26,
    133–41
  health care and, 139–41
  home care in, 137–39
  incidence of, 19
  most common type of, 19–20
  parents and, *see* parents of
    leukemic children
  preventive radiotherapy in, 106,
    107–8
  sources of information on,
    131–32
  survival rates in, 1
chloramphenicol-induced acute
    myelocytic leukemia, 70
chromosomes
  DNA in, 31
  genetics and, 28
  See also Philadelphia chromo-
    some
chronic hepatitis, 66
chronic leukemias, treatment of,
    80–81
chronic lymphocytic leukemia, 17
  incidence of, 20
chronic myelocytic leukemia, 17,
    21–22
circadian rhythms, chemotherapy
    effectiveness and, 189–91
circulatory systems, leukemia and,
    4
clinical research, 157–58
cloning, 166
complement, 57–58
  immune response and, 13
computers
  designing drugs with, 191–92
  for selection of cancer treatment
    centers, 127n–28n
congenital chromosomal defects,
    susceptibility to leukemia and,
    70–71
constipation, 139–40
corticosteroids, white blood cells
    and, 57
costs, 130–31
  synthetic genes and, 166
counseling, sources of, 230–31
cytokines, 171

defective cells, phagocytosis and, 11
deoxynucleotidyl transferase pre-
    diction of relapse and, 154–55
deoxyribonucleic acid. *See* DNA
diarrhea, 144
diet
  as "cures," 147
  in Laetrile study, 148
  for leukemic children, 139–40
  loss of appetite and, 144
  prior to allogenic bone marrow
    transplantation, 114
DiGuglielmo's disease. *See* erythro-
    leukemia
DNA
  mutation, *see* mutation
  RNA and, 30
  RNA viruses and, 52
  structure and function of, 30
  viruses and, 49
  See also genetics research
DNA codes, applications of, 33–34
DNA damage
  causes of, 37–38
  leukemia and, 71
  viral-oncogene theory of leukemia
    and, 50–52
DNA repair, 38
  "cancer families" and, 40–41
  faulty, leukemia and, 75–76
  hereditary diseases and, 38
DNA viruses, 53–55
  See also herpes viruses
donor, of allogenic bone marrow,
    112–13
Down's syndrome
  genetic defect in, 36
  leukemia and, 70
drug research
  anti-cancer drugs and, 192–93
  approaches to, 190–91
  cell kinetics and, 186–93
  computers and, 191–92
  See also drugs
drugs
  anti-herpes, 104, 196–97
  clinical trials of, 186–88
  effectiveness of, 188
  hyperthermia and effectiveness
    of, 189
  synthesized by microorganisms,
    165–69

tests of, 157–58
ultrasound and effectiveness of,
    188
See also anti-leukemic drugs;
    chemotherapy; maintenance
    drugs

elderly
    chronic lymphocytic leukemia in,
        21
    leukemia incidence in, 2
electron microscopy, diagnosis of
    leukemia and, 25
enzymes
    DNA repair and, 38
    produced by RNA virus
        oncogenes, 49
    See also deoxynucleotidyl
        transferase
eosinophilic leukemia, 18
Epstein-Barr virus (EBV), 53–54
erythrocytes
    in acute myelocytic leukemia, 21
    development and function of, 8
    transfusions during chemotherapy,
        99, 100
erythroleukemia, 18

families, viral role in leukemia and,
    52
    See also "cancer families"
Fanconi's syndrome, leukemia and,
    70
Federal Drug Administration
    ban on Laetrile, 148–50
    drug approval by, 158
"fetal" proteins as malignancy-
    associated markers, 154
financial aid, sources of, 130,
    229–30
financial problems, 143
folic acid, white blood cells and,
    57
foreign cells, phagocytosis and, 11

gastrointestinal system, lymphoid
    tissue in, 15
gene mapping, genetic defects and,
    37
genes
    abnormalities in leukemia patients,
        15

carcinogens and, 41–42
    function of, 31–33
    leukemia research and, 73
    structure and function of, 28–35
    synthetic, *see* gene splicing
    virus, 42
    See also "cancer genes"; DNA;
        genetic defects
genetic code, 33
genetic damage, causes of, 37–38
    See also DNA damage
genetic defects, hereditary diseases
    and, 36
    See also "cancer families"
genetic engineering, 160–65
    interferon and, 172
    potential medical applications,
        165–69
    production of synthetic substances
        and, 165–67
    restrictions on, 164–65
genetics
    immune response and, 65–67
    normal cell differentiation and,
        2–3
genetics research, 159–67
    See also genetic engineering
genital herpes, 196–97
glycoproteins, white blood cells and,
    57–58
graft-versus-host-disease (GVHD)
    allogenic bone marrow transplan-
        tation and, 109, 113, 115–16
    autologous bone marrow trans-
        plantation and, 119
    treatment of, 115–16, 117
granulocytes, 11–13
    acute myelocytic leukemia and,
        21
    granulopoietin-stimulated produc-
        tion, 177
    transfusions in chemotherapy
        patient, 100
granulopoietin, 177
Graves's disease, 66

hair loss from chemotherapy, 98
hairy-cell leukemia, 18
harringtonin, 187
heart failure, ABMT and, 115

hemoglobin
 function of, 8
 sickle-cell anemia and, 36
hereditary diseases
 cancers associated with, 154
 genetic defects and, 36
 leukemia risk and, 40, 70–71
 vulnerability to cancer and, 74
herpes virus
 cancer and, 53–54
 immune-suppressed leukemia
  patients and, 104
 infections after ABMT and, 116
 leukemic children and, 140
 protection against, 195–96
 See also Epstein-Barr virus
histiocytic leukemia. *See* monocytic
  leukemia
Hodgkin's disease, 22–23, 66
hormonal imbalances, blood cells
  and, 5
hormones, anti-leukemia, 87
hospitals, NCI-associated, 129
 See also treatment centers
hydrocarbons, leukemia and, 70
hypersensitivity, 60
hyperthermia, 189

immune response system
 acute lymphocytic leukemia in
  children and, 72
 antigens and, 58–60
 B cells and, 14–15
 blood system and, 4–5
 chemotherapy and, 78–79, 103–4
 erythrocytes and, 8, 55–60
 genes in MHC region and, 65–67
 leukemia and, 76–77
 leukemia cells and, 4, 16, 67–70
 macrophages and, 12–13
 malignant cells and, 3, 27
 mechanical defenses, 55
 pharmacology and, 186–93
 primary and secondary responses,
  59–60
 scheme of, 60–64
 viruses and, 42–43
 white blood cells, 56–58
 See also immunology and immunotherapy; phagocytosis
immunoglobulin G deficiency, 72

immunoglobulins, 60
 See also antibodies
immunology and immunotherapy,
  79, 120–24, 169–85
 biological response modifiers,
  170–77
 monoclonal antibodies and,
  180–85
 vaccination with leukemic cells,
  177–80
inductive event in two-step theory
  of cancer, 73–75
infections
 blood cells and, 5
 chemotherapy and, 99–100
 DNA damage and, 37
 inflammation and, 8, 10
 lymphocytes and, 15
 See also opportunistic infections
infectious mononucleosis
 differentiation from leukemia,
  23–24
 Epstein-Barr virus and, 53–54
inflammatory response, 8, 10
inherited diseases, MHC antigens
  and, 66–67
interferons, 79
 as biological response modifiers,
  171–75
 herpes infections and, 104, 197
 immune response and, 13
 side effects of, 174
 viral infections and, 195–96
 white blood cells and, 57
ionizing radiation
 DNA damage and, 37
 -induced leukemia, 70
isolation, chemotherapy and,
  99–100

juvenile-onset diabetes, 66

kidneys
 bone marrow transplantation and,
  115
 uric acid formation in chemotherapy and, 101
Krebiozen, 147

Laetrile, 147–52
leukemia
 bibliography on, 235–38

clustering of cases of, 71–72
description of, 1
development of, 75–76
diagnosis of, 16–17, 23–26
DNA research and, 35–36, 73
as form of cancer, 4
identification of malignant white
    cells in, 10
immune system and, 76–77
incidence of, 1–2
linked diseases, 22–23, 40–41
mortality from, 1–2
overview of, 15–26
production of leukemic cells and,
    15–16
research in, *see* research
sources of counseling on, 230–31
susceptibility factors, 70–71
symptoms of, 23
treatment for, *see* treatment of
    leukemia
types of, 16–22
viral-oncogene theory of, 50–52
viruses and, 52–55
See also cancer; childhood
    leukemia; *and specific types of*
leukemia cells
anti-leukemia drugs and, 85
immune response and, 67–70
origin of, 27–28
production of, 15–16
"resting," chemotherapy and,
    80–81, 93
vaccination with, 177–80
leukemia patients
"desperation cures" and, 147–52
emotional reactions of, 125–26
financial aid for, 130, 229–30
medical costs of, 130–31
optimal treatment centers for,
    127–30
organizations for, 234
parenthood and, 195
sources of information for,
    131–33
transportation for, 232–34
See also adult leukemia patients;
    childhood leukemia
leukemia research. *See* research
Leukemia Society of America, 130
leukocytes, 5, 10
lithium carbonate, 102, 121–22

as biological response modifier,
    176–77
liver damage, chemotherapy and, 97
lungs, lymphocytes in, 15
lupus erythematosus, 60, 66, 70
lymph nodes, 4, 5, 15
lymph system, 5–6
immune responses and, 58
lymphocytes, 8, 9
Epstein-Barr virus and, 53–54
macrophages and, 12–13
malignant lymphomas and, 22–23
production and function, 13–15
See also B cells; NK cells; T cells
lymphoid line of leukocytes, 9, 10
lymphoid organs. *See* lymph nodes;
    lymph system
lymphoid stem cells, 13
in acute lymphocytic leukemia,
    19–20
lymphoid tissue, 15
See also Hodgkin's disease; ma-
    lignant lymphomas
lymphokines, 121, 171
See also interferons

macrophages, 11–13
Magnetrode, 189
maintenance drugs, 20
major histocompatibility complex
    (MHC), 65
Make Today Count, 131, 150–51,
    233
malignant cells
cell-surface markers on, 66–67
culture of, 188
Epstein-Barr virus and, 54
functions of, 3
immune response system to, 27,
    67–70
macrophages and, 13
NK cells and, 15
origin of, 27–28
phagocytosis and, 11
T cells and, 14
malignant lymphomas, 22–23
marijuana, 145
mast cell leukemia. *See* basophilic
    leukemia
medical centers. *See* treatment
    centers

MEDLARS computer system, 127n-28n
megakaryocytes, 8, 10, 22
megakaryocytic leukemia, 18, 22
Mendelian inheritance patterns, 65–66, 74, 158
MER vaccine, 120–21
MHC-antigen matching, 65–66
 blood donations and, 101–2
 improvements in, 117
 transplants and, 108–9, 111–12
MHC antigens, diseases linked to, 66
mitosis inhibitors, 87–88
mixed-cell leukemia, 18
mongolism. *See* Down's syndrome
monoclonal antibodies, 79, 117
 leukemia research and, 180–85
monocytes, 11–13
monocytic leukemia, 18, 22
mood elevators, 144–46
mortality, in leukemia, 1–2
 See also survival rates
multiple myeloma, 22
multiple sclerosis, 60
mutations
 in allogeneic bone marrow transplantation cells, 118
 carcinogens and, 41–42
 chemotherapy-induced, 96–97
 in two-step theory of cancer, 74
 leukemia and, 76
 viral in animals, 43–48
myasthenia gravis, 60, 66
myeloid line white blood cells. *See* phagocytes
myeloid stem cells, 8–11
 radiotherapy and, 107
myelomonocytic leukemia, 18

National Cancer Institute, 127, 129, 145, 170–71, 195
 Laetrile studies of, 147–48
"natural killer" lymphocytes. *See* NK cells
neutrophilic leukemia, 18
NK cells, 15, 75
nucleotides, 28–29
 structure of, 33
"null" cell leukemia. *See* undifferentiated leukemia

oncogenes, 47–48
"opportunistic" infections, 102–4
oxygen, erythrocytes and, 8
oxygen depletion, 7, 8

pain, drugs used for, 144–46
parents of leukemic children
 emotional responses of, 133–34
 health care responsibilities of, 139–41
 national organizations for, 233–34
 relapses and, 141
 residences for, 130, 232
 sources of information for, 127, 131–32
 treatment of child and, 134–37
pathogens, 11, 56
 See also bacteria; viruses
patient care. *See* leukemia patients
PDQ, 127n–28n
phagocytes, 11
phagocytosis, 11
phenothiazine, 145
phenylbutazone-induced leukemia, 70
Philadelphia chromosome, 21, 154
plasma, 5
plasma-cell leukemia, 19
plasmids, 162, 164
platelets, 5
 chemotherapy and, 97–98
 clumping, 101
 leukemic cells and, 16
 production of, 8, 10
 transfusion of, 100–101
pluripotent stem cell, 7, 16
polymorphocytic leukemia, 19
pregnancy, chemotherapy and, 98, 195
progenitor cells. *See* stem cells
promotional events in two-step theory of cancer, 73–75
promyelocytic leukemia, 19
prostaglandins, 13, 57
proteins
 amino acids and, 30–31
 malignancy and, 35–36
 produced by "cancer genes," 155
 See also antigens; complement
protocols for leukemia treatment, 82–83
pseudoenzymes, anti-leukemia, 89

psychotherapy for adult leukemia
    patients, 146

radiation
    cancer and, 44
    leukemia and, 70, 71
    RNA viruses and, 46–47
    two-step theory of cancer and, 74
    See also X-rays
radiation therapy. *See* radiotherapy
radiotherapy, 79, 105–8
    effectiveness determination,
        106–7
    side effects of, 107–8
    total-body, 112
recombinant DNA technology. *See*
    genetic engineering
red blood cells. *See* erythrocytes
Reiter's syndrome, 66
relapses, 123–24
    early indications of, 154–55
    in leukemic children, 141
remissions, 122–23
    in acute lymphocytic leukemia,
        20
    in acute myelocytic leukemia, 21
    allogenic bone marow transplants,
        110
    chemotherapy induced, radio-
        therapy and, 105
    chronic myelocytic leukemia and,
        21–22
    induction and maintenance of, 79
    optimal treatment centers and,
        127
    treatment of child in, 138
"rescue" therapy, toxic effects of
    chemotherapy and, 93
research, 153–96
    basic and clinical, 156–58
    "cancer genes," 155
    chemotherapy, 193–95
    investigational protocols and, 83
    prediction of chemotherapy
        response, 156
    protection against viral infections,
        195–96
    updates on, 236–37
    See also drug research; genetics
        research; immunology and
        immunotherapy; virology

residences for parents of leukemic
    child, 130, 232
restriction enzymes, 161–62
rheumatoid arthritis, 60
ribonucleic acid. *See* RNA
Rieder cell leukemia, 19
RNA, 30, 164
RNA tumor viruses, 42, 44, 45–48
    "cancer-genes" and, 48–52
    enzymes produced by, 49
    human leukemia and, 52–55
    interferon and, 172–73

sarcoidosis, 66
sedatives, 144–46
sensitization, donor blood products
    and, 104–5
serotonin, inflammatory response
    and, 8, 10
serum. *See* plasma
sexual problems of adult leukemia
    patients, 143
siblings of leukemic child, 137
sickle-cell anemia, 36
side effects
    of allogenic bone marrow trans-
        plantation, 118–19
    of antibiotics, 105
    of chemotherapy, 96–98
    handling, 144
    of interferon, 174
    of radiotherapy, 107–8
    of supportive therapy, 104–5
spinal fluid, chemotherapy and, 94
spleen, 4–5
stem-cell leukemia, 19
stem cells
    blood cell development and, 7–8
    induction of production of, 102
    lithium-stimulated production of,
        176–77
    normal vs. malignant, 119
    suppressive action of leukemia
        cells on, 16
sterility, chemotherapy and, 98
sunlight, DNA damage and, 37, 38
supportive therapy, 98–105
    objectives of, 78–79
    problems with donor blood
        products, 101–2
    side effects of, 104–5

surgery, 79
survival rates for leukemia, 1
  See also mortality

T cells, 13–14
  antigens and, 58–59
  growth factor and macrophage
    factor, 17
thymosin, 175–76
thymus, leukemic cells in, 4
tobacco smoke carcinogens
  cancer and, 41
  DNA mutation and, 154
toxic substances
  blood cells and, 5
  cancer susceptibility and, 41
  marrow stem cells and, 7
toxicity
  allogenic bone marrow trans-
    plantation and, 114–15
  of chemotherapy, 93
tranquilizers, 144–46
transplantation. *See* allogenic bone
    marrow transplantation; auto-
    logous bone marrow transplan-
    tation
transportation, 232–33
treatment centers, 227–29
  optimal, 127–130
treatment of leukemia, 78–124
  desperation "cures" and thera-
    pies, 147–52
  effectiveness of, 81
  facilities for, 117–19
  impact on cancer research, 81–82
  individual differences in, 80
  protocols for, 82–83
  remission and relapse, *see* re-
    lapse; remission
  research and, *see* research
  side effects of, 144
  support therapy, 78–79
  surgery and, 79
  See also bone marrow transplants;
    chemotherapy; immunotherapy;
    Laetrile; radiotherapy; research;
    supportive therapy
tumors
  carcinogen and radiation-induced,
    43

  growth of, 3
  malignant lymphomas and, 22–23
two-step theory of cancer, 73–75
  leukemia and, 16

ultrasound, drug effectiveness and,
    188
undifferentiated leukemia, 19
uric acid formation, chemotherapy
    and, 101
urinary problems, 144

vaccinations
  against herpes, 197
  antibodies and, 15
  leukemic cells, 177–80
  for leukemic children, 140
venereal herpes, cancer and, 54
viral oncogenes, 47–48
virology research, 185
viruses
  cancer-causing genes and, 42–55
  in bone marrow transplants, 118
  interferon and, 172–74
  leukemic children and, 140
  phagocytosis and, 11
  See also pathogens; RNA-tumor
    viruses
vitamin A, 57, 176
vitamins as antioxidants, 192–93

white blood cells
  distinguishing different types of,
    10
  function of, 5
  in leukemia, 1, 16, 23–24
  as regulatory agents, 56–58
  "teaching" systems for, 121
  transfusions during chemotherapy,
    99
  types of, 11–13
  See also granulocytes; leukocytes;
    macrophages; monocytes;
    myeloid white blood cells

X-rays
  DNA damage and, 37
  leukemia and, 70–71
xeroderma pigmentosum (XP), 38

Zovirax, 196–97